Sport and Physical Activity for Mental Health

Sport and Physical Activity for Mental Health

David Carless
*Carnegie Research Institute,
Leeds Metropolitan University, UK*

and

Kitrina Douglas
University of Bristol, UK

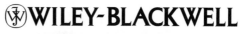

A John Wiley & Sons, Ltd., Publication

Library of Congress Cataloging-in-Publication Data

Carless, David, 1970–
Sport and physical activity for mental health / David Carless and Kitrina Douglas.
p. ; cm.
Includes bibliographical references and index.
ISBN 978-1-4051-9785-4 (pbk. : alk. paper)
1. Sports–Psychological aspects. 2. Exercise–Psychological aspects.
3. Mental illness–Exercise therapy. 4. Recreational therapy. I. Douglas, Kitrina. II. Title.
[DNLM: 1. Mental Disorders–rehabilitation. 2. Exercise–psychology.
3. Exercise Therapy–methods. 4. Occupational Therapy–methods.
5. Sports–psychology. WM 140 C278s 2010]
GV706.4.C363 2010
612′.044–dc22
2010001829

A catalogue record for this book is available from the British Library.

Set in 10/12 pt Sabon by Aptara® Inc., New Delhi, India
Printed and bound in Singapore by Ho Printing Singapore Pte Ltd

1   2010

Contents

Acknowledgements

While ours are the names on the front cover, this book would not have been possible without the investments, contributions, knowledge and support of many other people. We are indebted to the individuals who, in the course of being participants in our research, shared with us stories of their experience. For some, sharing these stories was not an easy process – it required strength, courage, trust and a generosity of spirit which we admire and respect. We thank all those individuals whose experiences and insights underpin this book yet who, for ethical regulations concerning anonymity of research participants, we are unable to mention by name. We would also like to acknowledge and thank several colleagues and friends who, in various ways, have generously contributed towards or supported our work: Laura Bennett, Ken Fox, Margot Hodgson, Jim McKenna, Brett Smith, David Stacey, Brendan Stone and Gerry Turvey.

Finally, we would like to acknowledge and thank three academics, writers and thinkers whose work has profoundly influenced the directions that we have taken in this book. In the field of counselling and psychotherapy, Kim Etherington's work exemplifies an approach and ethos to which we aspire. Kim's written work and the personal support she has offered have helped us to feel confident in pursuing a narrative direction. In the field of psychology, the pioneering work of Peter Chadwick has provided an alternative vision for what psychology could be and has simultaneously generated unique insights into the nature of psychotic experience. Through his work and personal communications, Peter has encouraged us in our work while provoking us to reflect on our own perspectives and ways of working. Within the field of sport and physical activity, the work of Andrew Sparkes has consistently broken new ground in the areas of qualitative research, narrative inquiry and creative methods. Without the solid foundation and the inspiration that Andrew's work has provided – not to mention the personal support and encouragement he has offered us both over the years – this book would never have got off the ground.

David Carless and Kitrina Douglas

Credits

Introduction

This book is about physical activity, sport and mental health. More specifically, the book is an exploration of the ways in which various forms of physical activity and sport contribute to recovery among people who have at some time in their life been diagnosed with a mental illness. Our focus is therefore directed primarily towards the lives of people who have personally experienced mental health problems and are themselves involved in some kind of sport or physical activity.

We have two broad aims for the book, the first of which is to shed some new light on the processes by which physical activity and sport can contribute to recovery. Our interest here is less to do with answering the question *What effect does sport/physical activity have on mental illness?* and more to do with exploring the question *What does sport/physical activity mean for you in the context of your life?* To answer this question it is necessary to take seriously the stories individuals tell about their experiences because these stories reveal how they make sense of their lives (in relation to the past, present and future) and the place they give to physical activity and sport across their lives. If physical activity and sport are to be useful, inclusive and empowering activities for people with mental health problems then this kind of understanding is vital.

Our second aim is to generate some insights regarding the kinds of physical activity and sport opportunities that are most likely to be experienced as 'useful' by individuals with mental health problems. Our interest here is of a practical nature in that we seek to shed light on the ways in which physical activity and sport opportunities may be successfully initiated, offered and supported in mental health contexts.

Throughout the book we have tried to provide information and material which will stimulate informed reflection among those who are involved with or interested in physical activity and sport provision. In this sense, the book offers a reservoir of resources, provocations and insights which we hope will encourage you – whether you are a practitioner, student or researcher – to reflect on your own ideas and approaches in the context of your particular interests.

The narrative approach that we utilise throughout the book is oriented towards an appreciation that what is needed at this point in time is not so much more *facts* (i.e. propositional forms of knowledge concerning *what we know*), but rather some different kinds of understanding which provide guidance concerning *what to do with what we know*. As Arthur Frank (2000 a, p. 363) has put it, at this point in history 'more knowledge may be less important than a clearer sense of value … Deciding what to do about what we know requires having an ethical standpoint.' The kinds of understanding that we focus on in this book, we hope, provide an ethical basis for action within the many diverse contexts of physical activity, sport and mental health.

In an effort to achieve these aims in a way that is both accessible and intuitive, we have organised the book into three parts. In Part I, we set the scene by providing a theoretical and methodological backdrop. In chapter 1, we consider the experience of mental health problems, the processes of recovery and existing research in the field of physical activity and mental health. Highlighting what is missing from existing research leads us in chapter 2 to an explicit examination of our own approach – in terms of both theories and methods – towards the research which forms the foundations of the book.

In Part II our focus is on understanding – trying to make sense of – the physical activity and sport experiences of people who have been diagnosed with a mental illness. In chapter 3, we focus on two life stories which provide revealing insights into the personal nature of experiences of sport, physical activity and mental health. Our aim in this chapter is to open the door to possibilities and sow the seeds for a broad-based and holistic understanding of the ways in which human beings can experience mental health change through participation. In chapters 4 through 6, we withdraw from these stories to suggest three roles which sport and physical activity can play in recovery. In chapter 4 we explore how identity can be damaged through the experience of mental illness and how, for those individuals who hold an athletic identity, a return to meaningful sport or exercise participation can be an effective way to rebuild one's identity. In chapter 5 we explore how group-based forms of sport and physical activity can provide an opportunity for individuals to re-story their lives through creating and sharing action, achievement and relationship stories. Through these processes, we suggest, valuable and important aspects of recovery and personal redevelopment can be achieved. In chapter 6 we consider the ways in which sport and physical activity can act as a 'vehicle' or 'stepping stone' towards recovery through providing a number of outcomes which some people experience as beneficial.

Part III focuses on knowledge and understanding concerning effective and beneficial provision of sport and physical activity opportunities in mental health contexts. We draw on our research over the past decade in an effort to identify some strategies and approaches which enable practitioners to tailor 'the sport and exercise experience' in ways that are most likely to be experienced as beneficial. In chapter 7, we turn our attention to the cultural settings in which physical activity and sport take place. Socio-cultural factors inevitably influence the kinds of experience that individuals have through sport and exercise participation and, through being aware of these, practitioners will be better placed to offer beneficial and positive opportunities. In chapter 8 we focus on the needs of women in sport and physical activity to consider the reasons why large numbers of women may be disinclined towards sport and physical activity, and what can be done to improve provision for these women.

In chapter 9 we focus specifically on the provision of effective social support for people who are both initiating and maintaining sport or physical activity participation. In this chapter we identify four distinct forms of social support and consider how these forms might be facilitated in practice. In chapter 10 we draw on the expertise and knowledge of practitioners who have been involved in physical activity or sport provision in mental health settings. Through presenting conversations between ourselves and three practitioners we hope to stimulate ideas and approaches through reflecting on practical experiences of provision. In chapter 11 we share a story from our own practice which begins to tie together some of the diverse strands and concepts which have emerged throughout the book. The story draws attention to some of the possibilities and problems of physical activity and sport in mental health contexts in a way that is firmly rooted in day-to-day experience. Finally, in chapter 12, we offer our own interpretation and ideas concerning the ways in which research and practice in this field might be developed and extended in the coming years. We hope that this 'conclusion' of sorts will stimulate others to continue and refresh their ongoing efforts.

Part I

Setting the scene

A background to mental health and physical activity

Experiencing mental health problems

When Neil Armstrong set foot on the moon and spoke the legendary words, 'This is one small step for man, one giant leap for mankind,' his actions embodied the technological advances of his time. Donned in a space suit protecting him from a hostile environment, Armstrong's walk on the moon also symbolised, in many ways, that while science may have made significant breakthroughs, there is still so much we don't know, can't change or control. This is not only with regard to outer space and the planetary constellations that surround us. The space within *us* – physical, psychological, emotional and spiritual – remains an elusive and fascinating area of exploration, and this is certainly the case as we seek to understand and sustain mental health.

For the teams of scientists that supported the *Apollo* trip, it was possible to record every minute detail of Armstrong's physiology. However, the data recorded by some of the most sensitive equipment known to humankind was unable to inspire generations of children because this data, though complex and comprehensive, could not communicate to us what it *felt like* walking on the moon. In contrast, when Armstrong said, 'It's really pretty up here,' those listening on earth began to get an understanding. Isn't it amazing with all the tasks this astronaut had to accomplish that he took time to view the heavens and comment on their beauty? NASA's aim, of course, was to put a man on the moon and bring him back safely. Their interest probably wasn't on how this individual would describe his experience of the trip. Being human, however, means that collecting facts and figures only represented part of the complex picture of the journey, and gaining a more complete understanding of this journey required Armstrong to describe his experience. Understanding how Armstrong gave meaning to his experiences might not have been essential to maintaining homeostasis, but it is essential if we are to understand the man and support other astronauts.

This kind of perspective informs our approach in the book: it is a perspective which recognises the difference between knowledge and wisdom. As Patricia Deegan (1996, p. 91) has observed in the context of mental health, 'most students emerge from their studies full of knowledge but they lack wisdom or the ability to see the form or essence of that which is'. Wisdom of this kind is fundamental to understanding how physical activity and sport can contribute to recovery among people experiencing mental health problems. For us, this understanding starts with *experience*. We want to explore the question: 'What is it like to experience physical activity and sport in the context of mental health?' We also want to begin to appreciate *meaning*: 'What does physical activity and sport mean to individuals living with mental distress?' Science's focus travelling deep into the brain with ever-more complex equipment, having a better grasp of the aetiology of mental health and looking for clues at a microbiological level, only provides part of the picture. At times, this focus can come to divert attention and interest away from the person and how he or she experiences the recovery process.

To start this opening chapter, we leave physical activity and sport aside to focus on mental health and illness. We want to focus initially on the question: 'What is it like to experience mental health problems?' To answer this question, the focus must be directed towards the individual, personal level. Some readers might be able to draw upon their own experiences of mental ill-health, but if you have no experience of mental illness the stories of people who have walked these particular paths can provide important insights. Either way, the following accounts hopefully begin to draw attention to the diverse nature of experiences of mental health difficulties.

Several books exist which are dedicated to presenting and exploring stories of the experience of mental illness (e.g. Karp, 1996; Davidson, 2003) and we recommend these sources as they provide more comprehensive collections than we are able to provide here. In addition to these books, several individuals who have themselves experienced forms of mental distress have written about their experiences and published their accounts in health or social science journals. It is these accounts that we draw on now to give a flavour of what it can be like to experience mental health problems. We present below brief excerpts from the stories of three individuals: Peter Chadwick (2001a), Brett Smith (1999), and Stuart Baker-Brown (2006). Other examples can be found in the work of Patricia Deegan (1996) and Brendan Stone (2009).

> Alas there's no privacy here . . . no privacy anywhere . . . the cracks in the wall plaster . . . hidden microcameras in them . . . the walls, people listening, *listening* through them, like they did in Bristol, all the time. The window . . . binoculars on it, cameras with zoom lenses . . . they can see me . . . people watching, watching. The world a prison wherever I go. Horror behind, terror in front . . . but what do they want of me?! Are they trying to puncture my pathetic bloated ego with their pranks, as Sherwin used to do at school? Teach me a lesson? Cure me of my evil sensuous ways? Make me 'come down'? Under observation, always under observation . . .
>
> But there's a knock on the door. It'll be Tony McAdam from downstairs. It is. He asks if I have any cigarettes. I say no. Tell him I've given up smoking, which I have. He launches into (yet another) anecdote about how he beat up this guy the previous night. I say quickly, 'Ooooh, fighting, even more frightening than homosexuality!'

He looks at me slightly surprised. I notice for the first time that I sound mad. What a thing to say. I really do, I really sound mad . . .

What a district this is. Hackney. How did I ever come to live here? Nowhere else in London will take you if you have a dog. You can't get a room anywhere. Certainly not in West London anyway. Everybody's business is everybody's business. No privacy, no-one has any loyalty anymore. Slagging people off, slagging people off, that's all it is . . . all the time. And I'm right in the middle of it. Transparent, invaded, betrayed. That's my life.

(Chadwick, 2001a, p. 55. Copyright © 2001, SAGE Publications.
Reproduced with permission.)

Upon pinching our pale skin, a barely audible question escapes from our mouth: 'How are we doing?'

Silence. We listen to our breathing – it is shallow and pathetic. 'Are we all right?' Slowly we shake our head. We don't want to speak – not today anyway.

'Morning,' we whisper. The word flickers in our consciousness. 'How are we feeling today?'

'Not the best,' is the apathetic reply. 'Today's going to be another bad one,' we say stoically.

We feel the violence of the vortex gather pace as it screams inside our body. We twist through its complexity and pound on our corporal self. As usual, questions concerning its authenticity bob up and down in our sea of pain. *How do we really feel? The word doesn't describe our feelings – does it? Surely it's unimaginable to those who have not suffered with it? People walking down the street, students, friends – whatever – nonchalantly spew it out. It seems that the word, like a slug slithering innocuously through language and culture, leaves little trace of its intrinsic malevolence. Has it become so common in everyday language? Has it lost its depth, its meaning, and its feeling? Has it been hammered into banality?* we think. As always, however, we struggle for answers while our mind becomes a cesspool of ominous thoughts. We become swamped in our(selves).

The torture continues in our head. How can life be filled with such torpid indifference? The little things like taking our dog for a walk in the park on a warm spring day or playing football with our friends just aren't fun anymore. We breathe and walk, we just don't live. We are detached and hollow. Under our blanket of suffocating darkness, we pretend that everything is fine, yet, we rot away from the inside. At times it spews bits out. At times it swallows us whole. At times both. No warning, bang! We move from pain to pain. We have only one future. Please God, help, we plead as our huddled body rocks back and forth.

Confused and afraid, we don't want to talk anymore. 'Please leave,' we gently sob.

(Smith, 1999, p. 264. Copyright © 1999, SAGE Publications. Reproduced with
permission.)

As I write these words, I can recall my paranoia and fear building up on a daily basis.

I tried to convince myself that I was under no threat and that my fears were unjustified, but I quickly began to be afraid of everyone and feared that my life was in danger. I did not know what to do. I had no idea that I could have paranoid schizophrenia; I did not even know what schizophrenia was.

Stress and paranoia began to take their toll. I quickly became confused in my thinking and obsessed that I was being followed. Often, when I got back to my bedsit after work I would huddle in the corner of the room in fear.

As the weeks passed and pressure took its toll, I had to take time off work. Anxiety and paranoia were now quickly and devastatingly beginning to run my life, and a deep-rooted illness was setting in.

During this time I had my first and worst psychotic experience. It was an extremely frightening time and still scares me now as I think of it. As I lay on my bed trying to relax, I suddenly found myself in complete darkness. I had the experience of being physically vortexed into my own dark mind. I cannot truly explain what went on, but the feeling of it still terrifies me. I screamed to be let out, and as I screamed I found myself back on my bed with a strange sensation around my head. It was as though I was sucked into my own dark mind away from any life or reality.

(Baker-Brown, 2006, p. 636. Copyright © 2006, BMJ Publishing Group Ltd. Reproduced with permission.)

On reading and re-reading these stories, we find ourselves reflecting on each individual's experiences, wanting to know more and wondering what happened next. We both feel a range of emotions as we read and reflect on the stories, which may resonate with or be initiated by the vivid descriptions within each account. While each of us responds to different details within the stories, feeling different emotions in different ways, we both find the stories difficult to read or hear – they are troubling and challenging, perhaps because of the degree of suffering they portray. There are some recurring themes which strike us in the stories: a strong sense of *fear*, how the experiences recounted were experienced as frightening or even terrifying; a sense of *isolation*, that the teller recounts feeling somehow separated or removed from other people and/or life; a sense of *joylessness*, a loss of fun, humour, enthusiasm; *hopelessness*, a loss of optimism or interest in the future; a loss of *agency* or autonomy, a feeling of being out of control; a sense of *inactivity*, inertia, feelings of nothingness or emptiness; and, finally, a sense that the experience of distress is *total*, complete and permeates across many aspects of the individual's life in profound ways.

For us, perhaps the most striking theme across the stories is their *diversity*. Although each story describes the experience of mental health difficulties, the stories are varied and individual both in terms of the particular events and actions recounted as well as the individual's emotional response to those occurrences. The themes we identify above arise from *our* perspective on the stories – we see the stories through the lens of our own experience. In recognition of this, and because the stories are so diverse and complex, we encourage you to reflect on the stories from *your* perspective in order to form your own interpretations and conclusions. What do *you* feel having read the stories? How would *you* respond to the experiences recounted in the stories? Our reason for presenting this selection of stories here and now is to allow for this openness, because we understand that mental health and illness can be experienced in many different ways which relate to individual circumstances, biographies, experiences and contexts. We hope that these brief passages provide some insights and provoke some reflection on what is clearly a very personal yet highly distressing and extremely difficult set of experiences.

Attendant to each story – either before or after the events recounted – is likely involvement with mental health services and, therefore, the medical processes of diagnosis and treatment. We would now like to briefly consider this aspect of experience by presenting a further story of one individual's contact with mental health services which is taken from the writings of Baker-Brown (2007), who was diagnosed with, and treated for, schizophrenia. A further and comparable example may be found in Deegan (1996):

> I was unprepared for the weeks after my diagnosis, during which my psychiatric nurse told me that it was very likely that 'I would never work again in my life' and that the rest of my life would probably be about 'fighting to keep my schizophrenia under control'. I had never contemplated not working again and had always assumed that I would gain control over my illness and one day, sooner rather than later, be able to return to work.
>
> These statements from my nurse threw me completely. More was to follow from the trust. My nurse told me that I had 'to prove' that I could function as a normal member of society and that I would not be 'a threat' to anyone. I was shocked by these words and this very poor attitude towards me and my illness. The demoralisation caused by my illness was complete, and soon after receiving my diagnosis I became a broken man. The trust's lack of proper care and understanding of my needs as a person with schizophrenia, and being treated more as a 'condition' that needed controlling than a person who needed 'understanding', made sure of that.
>
> (Baker-Brown, 2006, p. 637)

This account raises the important issue of how the processes of being diagnosed with and treated for a mental health problem can interact in powerful ways with a person's understanding of themselves and their goals and aspirations for life. While the previous stories of the experience of mental distress are diverse, varying widely in terms of both their form and content, accounts of what it is like to 'be a mental health patient' often exhibit a worryingly high level of agreement and consistency concerning the ways in which diagnosis and treatment can in themselves be a damaging experience. It seems to us that a two-level impact is described by many people who have written about mental illness: First, the experience of a mental health problem is in itself traumatic and potentially damaging. Second, the experiences accompanying diagnosis and treatment can – for some people – lead to a second level of trauma and suffering. One result of this can be the loss or denial of the day-to-day freedom and opportunities that many of us take for granted. In this regard, as Chadwick (1997b, p. 580) puts it, 'there is no doubt that a psychotic episode leads to severe marginalization, pejorative categorization and disempowerment'.

A conceptualisation of mental health

In light of these and many other diverse accounts of mental health and illness, what position might we take in terms of conceptualising or defining mental health and illness? While we are reluctant to prescribe a specific definition, a working conceptualisation seems necessary. We are drawn to the broad and humanistic definition of mental health provided by the Department of Health (2003) which states that mental health is 'the emotional and spiritual resilience which enables us to enjoy life and to survive pain, disappointment and sadness. It is a positive sense of well-being and an underlying belief in our own and others' dignity and worth' (p. 8). In the United States, a similarly broad definition of mental health is provided in the Surgeon General's Report which sees mental health as 'a state of successful performance of mental function, resulting in productive activities, fulfilling relationships with other people, and the ability to adapt to change and to cope with adversity' (US Department of Health and Human Services, 1999, p. 4).

Although we are cautious of using the terms 'illness' or 'ill-health' in the context of mental health on the basis of the adverse effects such labelling can have on individuals (see, for example, Rogers & Pilgrim, 2005), we find it difficult to talk about our research or describe our research participants' backgrounds and experiences without using these terms. This particularly applies to the terms *serious mental illness* and *severe and enduring mental illness* because they are routinely used to cover the variety of diagnoses which apply to the individuals with whom we have worked. So while we try to minimise our use of these potentially pejorative terms, when we do employ them we follow the definition of serious mental illness as 'a diagnosable mental disorder found in persons aged 18 years and older that is so long lasting and severe that it seriously interferes with a person's ability to take part in major life activities' (US Department of Health and Human Services, n.d.).

Another way of defining mental health and illness might be on the basis of its aetiology; however, this in itself is a highly contested area. Rogers and Pilgrim (2005) and Chadwick (2009) provide thorough discussions of recent and current debates concerning the causation of mental health and illness. As these authors make clear, arguments have raged over decades – and continue in some quarters – regarding the extent to which mental health is seen as biologically determined (through genetic makeup, for example) or shaped by socio-cultural, environmental, economic and psychological factors. With regard to this question, Rogers and Pilgrim (2005, p. 3) write:

> It may be argued that biological treatments that bring about symptom relief themselves point to biological aetiology ... However, this may not follow: thieving can be prevented quite effectively by chopping off the hands of perpetrators, but hands do not cause theft. Likewise, a person shocked following a car crash may feel better by taking a minor tranquillizer, but their state is clearly environmentally induced. The thief's hands and the car crash victim's brain are merely biological mediators in a wider set of personal, economic and social relationships.

We consider that, for a variety of reasons which recur throughout the book, mental health and illness are heavily shaped by a host of social, cultural, psychological, biographical and contextual factors. On this basis, we share the perspective that mental health is not determined by biological or biochemical factors, but that these factors act as mediators or vehicles for psychological changes. Although all psychological processes are, at the most fundamental level, carried out by biochemical or biological processes this does not imply that chemical or biological factors actually *caused* a particular disorder (Bedi, 1999). While some will beg to differ, either as proponents of biological and genetic determinism or supporters of a wholly socio-cultural explanation, our work has led us to accept Chadwick's assessment of current opinion regarding the causes of mental health problems. In his words:

> In light of the fact that the pendulum in research internationally has swung first from environmentalism ('mind with no brain') to biochemical reductionism ('brain with no mind'), it now rests pretty well between these misguided earlier extremes and both genetic and constitutional vulnerability as well as environmental and cognitive, emotional and motivational factors are recognised as important in explanation and recovery. (2009, p. x)

From this perspective, Chadwick identifies and expresses well a stance in relation to recent debates concerning the genetic determination of mental illness (in this case, schizophrenia) which aligns with our own perspective on mental health and illness. This conception seems to us to offer a constructive, ethical and humanistic way forward. As he explains, to understand the extent to which 'genetic vulnerability' influences the occurrence of mental health problems it is necessary to consider the role of many genes which each have, at best, only a small to moderate effect on mental health. These genes, he points out, are widely distributed in the population and are also likely to be associated with valuable qualities and abilities such as perceptual sensitivity, creative and linguistic imaginativeness and meaning-seeking. Hence, in Chadwick's words, 'we are all "a little schizophrenic", it is part and parcel of the human condition and may indeed *be* why we are such an imaginative and creative, inventive species' (2009, p. xi). Importantly, he points out:

> This conceptualisation of schizophrenia sees sufferers as kith and kin with the rest of humanity, sees madness as not essentially an alien state experientially but something that everybody, because of their humanity, has at least a slight inkling of at some time in their lives. Schizophrenia, in my view, and as a sufferer who has known it from the inside, is essentially an exaggeration of normal processes that interweave with toxic results for one's well-being and, on many occasions, for one's very willingness to stay alive at all. (p. xi)

This conception, we think, emphasises the core concept of humanity which we all share, and resists casting as 'Other' those who experience mental health problems by suggesting people who experience mental health problems are in some way 'different' from those who do not. By taking this perspective, we hope that our work contributes to an increased awareness of *similarity* and reduced perceptions of *difference* which help fracture damaging distinctions between 'them' and 'us'. This philosophy is critical to the work we describe in this book and central to the task of offering or supporting sport and physical activity opportunities which are likely to be experienced as helpful.

The concept of recovery

A notable shift has taken place in recent years within the mental health field in terms of what *recovery* is taken to entail. Julie Repper and Rachel Perkins (2003) note that the traditional focus of treatments and services for people with mental health problems has been on symptom alleviation – often through medication regimes – and suggest this has led to a culture within mental health services which is preoccupied with deficits and dysfunctions. Within this culture, these authors suggest, need is assessed in terms of symptoms to be alleviated, interventions are focused upon difficulties, and effectiveness is evaluated in terms of symptom removal or 'cure'. While modern treatments, very often medication, may be effective in symptom alleviation terms, those who have experienced mental illness often assert that elimination of symptoms is only one part of the recovery picture – that something more than the remission of symptoms is necessary for recovery to occur. Chadwick (1997a, p. 48), for example, recalls how 'despite the quite incredible power of the medication to wipe out symptoms (for which I will always be grateful) the inner feelings of downheartedness and guilt were still there'.

With a similar attention to a broader and more humanistic set of recovery-related factors, Repper and Perkins (2003, p. ix) write:

> The challenge facing people with mental health problems is to retain, or rebuild, a meaningful and valued life, and, like everyone else, to grow and develop within and beyond the limits imposed by their cognitive and emotional difficulties. Recovery is not about 'getting rid' of problems. It is about seeing people beyond their problems – their abilities, possibilities, interests and dreams – and recovering the social roles and relationships that give life value and meaning. This requires hope and opportunity. Building for a future necessitates a belief in the possibility of that future. Hope is the motivating force that gives life purpose and direction, but, without the opportunity to do the things you want to do, such hope is easily snuffed out.

In a similar vein, William Anthony (1993) describes recovery as a unique and personal process which involves a transformation of values, feelings, attitudes, goals, skills or life roles. In his words, it is 'a way of living a satisfying, hopeful, and contributing life even within the limitations caused by illness. Recovery involves the development of new meaning and purpose in one's life, as one grows beyond the catastrophic effects of mental illness' (1993, p. 19). From this perspective, the recovery process can be appreciated as far-reaching, complex and closely related to each individual's particular life experiences.

A very similar viewpoint has been reiterated more recently by Davidson and colleagues (2005) who, in attempting to establish a conceptual framework for recovery, argue that remission of symptoms or other deficits is not necessary for recovery. Rather, they suggest, 'recovery involves incorporation of one's illness within the context of a sense of hopefulness about one's future, particularly about one's ability to rebuild a positive sense of self and social identity' (2005, pp. 484–5). Rebuilding this sense of self and a social identity is also an important aspect of Davidson and Roe's (2007, p. 462) concept of *recovery in serious mental illness* (as opposed to recovery *from* mental illness) which they suggest is needed to overcome the 'loss of valued social roles and identity, isolation, loss of sense of self and purpose in life' which frequently accompanies severe mental health problems.

From the perspective of those who have experienced mental health problems, alleviation of symptoms is only one part of a more complex recovery picture. The recovery process, it seems, is likely to be unique to each individual and closely tied to situational and contextual factors as well as personal life experiences. It is on this basis that Coleman (1999) argues against defining recovery in terms of standardised outcome measures such as symptom rating scales and quality of life scales on the basis that they may hold little meaning for particular individuals and fail to allow for the personal and subjective nature of recovery. For us the priority is *meaning* over *measurement*. Instead of a set of tightly defined criteria through which recovery may be defined and measured, it seems more useful to conceptualise an open and loosely defined 'menu' of themes which hold meaning for the individual and are present across diverse conceptions of recovery. Core themes of recovery as identified by those who have themselves experienced mental illness (based on Anthony, 1993; Repper & Perkins, 2003; Davidson *et al.*, 2005) focus on the need to:

- rebuild social roles and relationships
- develop meaning and purpose in one's life
- recreate a positive sense of self and identity
- change one's attitudes, values and goals
- enact, acquire and demonstrate ability
- pursue personal interests, hopes and aspirations
- develop and maintain a sense of hopefulness about one's future.

Physical activity and mental health research

Over the past decade or so a handful of books have been published which have explicitly explored the relationships between physical activity and mental health through reviewing the existing research in the field. These include Morgan (1997), Biddle *et al.* (2000), Leith (2002) and Faulkner and Taylor (2005). In addition, several review articles have been published in academic journals and books during this time, some of which have focused on physical activity within the context of severe forms of mental illness. These include Faulkner and Biddle (1999), Fox (1999, 2000), Grant (2000), Carless and Faulkner (2003), Callaghan (2004), Richardson *et al.* (2005), Saxena *et al.* (2005), Faulkner and Carless (2006), Stathopoulou *et al.* (2006), Ellis *et al.* (2007) and Teychenne *et al.* (2008a). Numerous research papers have been published from the diverse perspectives of sport and exercise science, health promotion, mental health, nursing, psychology, public health and sociology. Published research studies over the past decade or so which have focused specifically on physical activity and sport within the context of severe and enduring forms of mental illness include Faulkner and Sparkes (1999), Raine *et al.* (2002), Carter-Morris and Faulkner (2003), Crone *et al.* (2004), Jones and O'Beney (2004), Beebe *et al.* (2005), Fogarty and Happell (2005), Skrinar *et al.* (2005), McDevitt *et al.* (2006), Crone (2007) and Soundy *et al.* (2007). Finally, several studies drawn from our own ongoing research (which forms the basis of this book) have been published: Carless and Douglas (2004, 2008a, 2008b, 2008c, 2008d, 2009c), Carless (2007, 2008) and Carless and Sparkes (2008).

A large volume of physical activity and mental health research has focused on exploring the relationship between participation and the occurrence of depression. Several reviews of this research have been published and authors of these papers report an inverse relationship between physical activity participation and the occurrence of depressive symptoms (e.g. Mutrie, 2000; O'Neal *et al.*, 2000; Lawlor & Hopker, 2001; Saxena *et al.*, 2005; Stathopolou *et al.*, 2006; Teychenne *et al.*, 2008a). At the population level, there is evidence that people who are physically active are less likely to experience depression (e.g. Teychenne *et al.*, 2008b) while among groups of people who are experiencing clinical depression, physical activity leads to statistically significant reductions in scores on symptom rating scales (e.g. Stathopolou *et al.*, 2006). The positive effects of various forms of physical activity on depression are now widely recognised and acknowledged in the Chief Medical Officer's Report (Department of Health, 2004) which recommends exercise as a treatment and preventive measure against depression.

It is evident that the majority of research conducted to date – and reviews of that research – have tended to focus primarily or exclusively on the extent to which physical activity alleviates the symptoms of mental health problems. For example, in reviewing the research which has explored the therapeutic potential of exercise for people with schizophrenia, Faulkner (2005) considers the potential psychological effects of exercise exclusively in terms of the alleviation of positive and negative symptoms. A similar symptom-focused orientation is evident in the review by Ellis and colleagues (2007) concerning the therapeutic effects of exercise among people with psychosis. In this regard Crone and colleagues (2005, p. 601) observe that 'researchers have concentrated on establishing a relationship, rather than asking why a particular incident, experience or situation is important'. By focusing on *measurement* (i.e. measuring what activity 'takes away' in terms of symptoms, impairments or problems) as opposed to *meaning* (i.e. understanding what activity contributes or brings to a person's life), the ways in which physical activity and sport may help individuals recover from mental health problems have mostly been sidelined. These include the possibility of changing attitudes, values, feelings, goals, skills and/or roles or providing a way to live a satisfying, hopeful and contributing life. Focusing on what activity *removes* as opposed to what it *contributes* is, we think, an important and significant oversight because, as Anthony (1993, p. 20) suggests:

> efforts to positively affect the impact of severe mental illness can do more than leave the person less impaired, less dysfunctional, less disabled, and less disadvantaged. These interventions can leave a person with not only 'less', but 'more' – more meaning, more purpose, more success and satisfaction with one's life.

To date, it is evident that the literature on physical activity and mental health has largely failed to address the potential for exercise and sport to contribute to recovery in this kind of broad, humanistic and positive sense.

It is notable that recent qualitative research which has focused on service-user perspectives on physical activity has tended to identify 'non-medical' kinds of benefits which are not necessarily related to mental health diagnosis or symptom occurrence. For example, Crone and Guy (2008) report a range of benefits as perceived by service users who participate in sports therapy activities. These included feelings of accomplishment and well-being, enhanced self-esteem, a more positive mentality, greater mental alertness, increased energy and improved mood. Similarly, Crone (2007) identifies several perceived benefits among members of a walking project which included enjoyment, opportunity to meet and be with people, knowledge and appreciation of plants, purposeful activity and help with sleeping.

Raine and colleagues (2002) note that not all therapeutic interventions aimed at relieving mental distress are equally valued by recipients and suggest that a critical factor in their value is the degree to which the intervention is seen as meaningful and relevant to a person's life. Clearly, meaning and relevance are highly subjective; what is meaningful and relevant to one person may be meaningless or irrelevant to another. From the perspective of researching the recovery process, developing an understanding of what is essentially a subjective process would seem to require a focus of attention on how individual persons experience recovery with reference to their own preferences, values and life circumstances.

According to Richardson and colleagues (2005), exercise is generally well accepted by people with serious mental illness and is often considered one of the most valued components of treatment among those who participate. On the basis of the Crone (2007) and Crone and Guy (2008) studies, it would seem that what users value most as outcomes from their physical activity and sport experiences has less to do with 'being a person with a mental illness' and more to do with 'being a human being'. In other words, research which takes as its starting point the voices of service users seems to us to point towards a need to consider the role of sport and exercise in a holistic and person-centred manner rather than in terms of symptom alleviation.

A final point which we would like to mention is that existing research in this field currently provides little theoretical insight into *how* mental health changes come about through involvement in physical activity. At present, there seems to be little understanding of possible *processes* of change. While this understanding need not be definitive, fixed, infallible or final, we do need some kind of lens through which to understand or 'make sense' of what happens when a person engages in sport or exercise. While some researchers strive for a biochemical explanation (for reviews of this work see Morgan, 1997), these approaches have so far failed to identify a single causative mechanism, perhaps because no single biochemical mechanism is responsible for the diverse range of effects which are possible through physical activity. What is needed, therefore, in order to complement existing knowledge in this area, is an alternative tack that can combine social, cultural and psychological approaches in order to provide insights into processes which, while perhaps involving biochemical change, cannot be reduced to biology or chemistry.

Key points

- Stories of the experience of mental health problems are highly diverse and individual. However, we see several themes (which may be experienced in different ways) across personal accounts of mental illness. These include fear, isolation, joylessness, hopelessness, a loss of agency, a sense of inactivity or emptiness, and distress that is total, permeating a person's life in profound ways.
- The experience of a mental health problem – alongside the processes of diagnosis and treatment – can interact in powerful ways with a person's understanding of themselves and their goals and aspirations for life. Often, people who have experienced severe mental health difficulties describe a loss of identity and sense of self alongside a loss of meaning and purpose in their lives. Marginalisation and disempowerment are common themes in individuals' accounts of being users of mental health services.

■   Recovery necessitates more than the alleviation of symptoms. It is widely recognised as a deeply personal and individual-specific process which is likely to include several tasks: rebuilding social roles and relationships; developing meaning and purpose in one's life; recreating a positive sense of self and identity; changing one's attitudes, values and goals; acquiring and enacting ability; pursuing personal interests, hopes and aspirations; developing and maintaining a sense of hopefulness about one's future.

■   Most existing research reports broadly positive conclusions regarding the mental health benefits of physical activity. However, the majority of studies have focused primarily on the potential of physical activity to alleviate symptoms as opposed to contributing to recovery in a broad and holistic manner.

■   The potential contribution of physical activity and sport in mental health may have more to do with what participation *contributes* to a person's life, rather than what it *takes away.*

A narrative approach to mental health research 2

You're looking at a person. There's quantitative bits of a person – height, weight – but then there's the 'How do they walk in?' 'Have they got a spark in their eye?' 'Are they looking you in the eye when you're talking?' All sorts of things are going on.

David Stacey (chapter 10)

In this chapter, we explore the narrative approach to mental health research that underpins this book. As we began to write, considering how best to describe the theories and methods that have guided our work, a friend and colleague, Brett Smith, invited us to respond to a research question he was investigating (see Smith, 2010). Brett's question was: *Why do scholars turn to narrative inquiry?* Brett and Andrew Sparkes – through their own research (e.g. Smith & Sparkes, 2002, 2004; Sparkes, 1996, 1998) and through informed discussions (e.g. Smith & Sparkes, 2005, 2006; Sparkes, 2000, 2008) – have been strong advocates for the use of narrative inquiry in the field of physical activity and sport. To answer Brett's question in the context of *our* experience, we both created a reflective text, David's a 1500-word first-person account commencing at the time of his PhD, and Kitrina's a 3000-word story commencing with her current interests.

Noticeable in our texts are different starting points, life events and styles of writing. As our writing in this book adopts a unified 'we', these differences are hidden. Alongside differences, we also noted comparable epiphanies in our stories which had caused each of us to feel tensions with, and ask questions about, traditional research methods. We both recount a degree of disillusionment with the scientific method when applied to people and their experience of their lives. These kinds of feelings are not unusual among narrative researchers (see, for example, Bochner, 1997; Etherington, 2004; Pelias, 2004; Clandinin & Murphy, 2007; Sparkes, 2007). Alongside these tensions were paradigm shifts in our understanding. Our accounts reveal how we each became uncomfortable with the assumptions underlying the positivist paradigm – in particular its mantra that in order to conduct robust research we must become detached and distanced and assume an unbiased and objective state. We both, for different reasons, experienced tensions when the literature that was informing our studies was challenged by what we experienced, or observed. We both asked the question: *Does it have to be like this?* For Alain de Botton (2000), whether it is for political reform or scientific development, dissatisfaction with how things are is a motivating force that drives change.

A word on reflexivity

In the context of the narrative research which forms the basis of this book, our own journeys towards narrative matter because *we* cannot be separated from the 'findings' we present. A recurring theme in feminist research has been how the relationship between researcher and subject is obscured through scientific methods. As Michelle Fine and colleagues (2000, p. 108) note, there has been a tendency to 'view the social science observer as a potential contaminant, something to be separated out, neutralised, minimised, standardized and controlled'. This stance represents an impossible aim which, as Ruth Behar (1993) explains, makes others vulnerable through positioning the researcher behind a cloak of alleged neutrality.

Instead, what we observe when we enter the research environment is that the re-lationships we form with participants and the types of questions we ask are filtered through the individual/s conducting the research. No individual can achieve neutrality or detachment because we all have pre-existing values and assumptions, a moral code and a way of being in the world. It is a little like suggesting that a tea bag immersed into boiling water will not have an effect on – and be affected by – what it has been plunged into. The world we are plunged into infuses our beings as we influence those around us. Our interpretation of everything we see, hear, say or touch has already been shaped by our education, family background, expectations, cultural norms, myths, and so on. These biases and assumptions are not in themselves inherently good or bad, but denying their existence – or giving the illusion that we can exist, as researchers, uncon-nected to the world and the people we research – can be damaging to the research, to our participants and to our own development as social beings.

One way to remove the cloak which shrouds research is to become a reflexive researcher who tries to bring a level of transparency to the research process. For Kim Etherington (2007a), reflexivity:

- diffuses through every aspect of the research process and challenges researchers to consider and address the ideology, culture, and politics of the participants and the potential audience of the research;
- is 'an ability to notice our responses to the world around us, to stories, and to other people and events, and an effort to use that knowledge to inform and direct our actions, communications and understandings' (p. 601);
- leads to an awareness of the personal, social and cultural contexts in which we are immersed and to an appreciation of how these contexts influence the conduct, interpretation and representation of research accounts.

In writing about the process of becoming a reflexive researcher, Etherington (2004) suggests that reflexivity should be seen as a work in progress, as something we strive towards which 'implies movement, agency and continuity' and 'is based upon the notion that we are constantly changing and developing our identities, and they are never fixed' (p. 15). In this book, we strive to draw attention to the ways *we* – as researchers – are tied to the interpretations we put forward regarding physical activity and mental health. As human and social science researchers, we inevitably find ourselves 'pointing at' participants – their lives and experiences. Through reflexive strategies we try to also 'point at ourselves' as we 'point at' the participants. To do so, we seek ways to:

- be transparent about our own ideology, culture and politics;
- show consideration of how power is unevenly distributed at different times during a research project and when representing findings;
- show *what* we know and *how we came to know*.

A problem we face is: by what means do we stand outside our embodied selves and our research practices to look at *our world* through a lens that brings transparency? Throughout this book we rely on a variety of approaches – including reflexive diaries (see Janesick, 2000), reflective interviews (this chapter and chapter 10), creative non-fiction (chapter 3) and fiction (chapter 11) – to bring a degree of transparency to our research. In the context of this chapter, Brett's question to us (Why did you turn to narrative inquiry?) provided the impetuous to move away from describing narrative theory and method in a distanced, impersonal way. Instead, it led us to reflect on *our own* journeys towards narrative. In the following section we hope to show – through an interview extract which focuses on David's journey[1] – *how* and *why* a narrative approach made sense, offered possibilities and hope, and brought clarity to this work. We hope that by choosing to use this strategy we set the tone for the book as a whole and move in the direction of transparency and reflexivity. By doing so we also hope to offer some solidarity to other researchers who may be struggling to make sense of their own data, research journey and ethical dilemmas.

A journey to narrative

Kitrina: David, I'd like to take you back to your first degree, can you remember why you used quantitative methods at that time?
David: I think I wanted neatness, I wanted answers, I wanted control, resolution, to solve things.
Kitrina: Do you remember what the results of your dissertation were?
David: I don't, apart from my advisor saying that the results didn't *prove* anything – that statistically speaking we couldn't say anything concrete because it was a small sample.
Kitrina: Then you started a Master's degree?

[1] We focus on David's journey for the purpose of illustrating the ways in which any researcher's background and experiences shape their research. This is not to say that Kitrina's journey is unimportant. Parts of Kitrina's journey to narrative have been published in Douglas (2009).

David: Yes, three years after finishing my first degree. And I did another quantitative thesis. I didn't really know anything about qualitative research at that time – it was allotted 2 hours out of 90 hours of research methods courses. The course was taught by a quantitative researcher and the way he portrayed qualitative research made it seem like it was just chatting to people. I was doing a Master's degree to get on, to get a decent job. I wasn't doing it because I was interested in it really, I just didn't hate it. Up to that point, I'd had a dozen jobs which I'd hated. I'd rather have been doing something else, but I could get a modest income through being a research and teaching assistant, and I didn't hate it. I *had* to get out of doing jobs I hated. So it was a case of, *you tell me what I have to do and I'll do it*. A quantitative study was a safe bet – I knew about those methods, it was what everyone seemed to be doing.

Kitrina: *And after your Master's you did your PhD, was that a career move?*

David: I was genuinely interested in physical activity and mental health – I'd found the area I was interested in and I read the books. But after studying the research papers and books, I kind of gave up believing research could tell us anything important about it. At the time there was very, very little research exploring physical activity and mental health in clinical populations, in contrast there was a lot of research with easy-to-access student groups – and it was all questionnaires. So, yes, it was just a job.

Kitrina: *How did doing your Master's influence your PhD?*

David: Well, I learnt from my Master's that I didn't want to stay in America and that on a day-to-day basis research was a damn sight better than the other jobs I'd had. I wasn't unhappy being a researcher, that's all I wanted, to not be unhappy in my work. It was a low goal but it had eluded me up to then. A PhD bursary gave me enough money to get by. I might have carried on doing research like that – where you don't really come into contact with the people you research – but because I couldn't get access to a mental health population at that time, a colleague suggested we use contacts in the department to study mental health and physical activity in a cardiac rehabilitation setting. I'd found a questionnaire I believed had potential, but it had over 200 items, so I realised the only way I was likely to get people to fill it in was to visit potential participants in hospital and ask them to help.

Kitrina: *So you only visited participants because you didn't think they would fill in the questionnaire otherwise?*

David: Yes. I didn't particularly want to do it, it was very labour intensive, I'd rather go for a surf or play my guitar. I didn't particularly want to go into a hospital, I don't particularly like hospitals.

Kitrina: *Your approach to research now appears radically different, is there something that brought about this change?*

David: Yes, it was the first time I'd been into a cardiac ward since I'd been in to visit my dad 3 or 4 years earlier. Suddenly, it brought back those feelings, it was: 'Hmmm, this is real people, and that was my dad in that bed, and this was us round that bed, visiting.' And it was quite traumatic for our family. So suddenly, it was very real to me, it wasn't *just* a research project any more. It made me think, this research doesn't really matter, in the greater scheme of things, compared to *that*. It's like – I need to *not* worry about recruiting participants. Someone has just nearly died. Faced by that situation it's almost impossible to push your research.

Kitrina: *But you did speak to them?*

David: Yes, I did, but I just tried to be a friend. Yes, I was trying to get data, but I thought I would just speak to them, introduce myself, have a conversation and explain what I was doing. But the ironic thing is, when you take that stance, people *want* to help. So they'd say, 'My wife's just coming in, could you come back in an hour', which I'd do, or they'd say, 'Yes sit down, what are you trying to do?' And then the question they all asked is, 'How will this help other people?'

Kitrina: *You felt very keenly from talking to them that they wanted to help other people?*

David: Yes, totally. I felt people were very vulnerable, they'd been shaken: life wasn't as secure as they thought it was. I suppose people had also received *care*. I remember my dad talked about the nurses and how wonderfully they looked after him, and maybe people want to pass that on. I got a really keen sense that people wanted to *contribute*. And I think for me, when faced with a person, an emotional body, I had to reappraise what was important to me. As soon as we started talking, these people invariably wanted, or needed, to talk about what had happened to them, and often he or she didn't have anyone to talk to. Family members can't be there all the time and anyway there are some things you can't talk to your family about. Everyone told me their stories.

Kitrina: *So how did that change you?*

David: I just felt there were so many insights and I was learning so much from what they were telling me. I can remember thinking: I wish people didn't have to go through such trauma to become humble. Or is it, like, only nice people have heart attacks? Are these just good people, caring people, or has their experience of illness made them that way? I'd started out in my Master's with, you know, *Does resistance training or aerobic exercise have a greater effect on mood*? But through the cardiac study I came to think those kinds of questions were – if not irrelevant – not that important to me.

Kitrina: *So would you say sitting on the side of the bed of someone who nearly died, and talking to them, changed the types of things you were interested in?*

David: Yes, I think it did. What they told me didn't affect my data, what we talked about *wasn't* my data. I was asking them to fill in a *questionnaire*. So the only information I analysed was what was on the questionnaire and all that they had said to me, those important insights, went in the bin. But when I looked at the data afterwards, compared to what they had been talking about, it seemed so superficial. It seemed I had binned all the really important stuff.

Kitrina: *So what did the data you had collected say?*

David: It stated the obvious really, it was very superficial. I thought, this isn't what matters, there's more, I am learning more from talking to people. There are things, very important things, that can't be *measured* – that can't be meaningfully represented by a number. Part of me accepted that if psychological research is about measuring people then that is what I must do. But part of me didn't.

Kitrina: *So what was the next change?*

David: I met a physio working in mental health and there was a chance to do some research there. I wanted to do that but there was also the time pressure of the PhD. So because I was radically shifting populations, I just thought *do the same thing* – in terms of the questionnaire approach – to give the PhD continuity, so it would 'pass'. It's people with severe and enduring mental health problems now, but the temperament and character inventory has been used a lot in psychiatric settings, so that's what I intended to do. But the consultant psychiatrist, while supportive of me doing some research, wouldn't allow me to use the questionnaire and he was on the ethics committee. So I had to rethink how I would approach the research.

Kitrina: Do you think that hearing the stories of cardiac patients had opened your eyes to a different way of doing research which made a difference at that moment?

David: Yes, if that hadn't happened, I might have given up and gone and looked for someone else to give a questionnaire to. It would have been an easier way to earn a PhD. But there was a beginning of a gut instinct, a feeling, that although I'm not interested or moved by the results of the questionnaire, I *was* interested in what people were telling me when I talked to them. I was in a department where everyone was an expert on research methods – but only from a positivistic perspective.

Kitrina: So you had very little knowledge of qualitative research?

David: Yes, I was scared to death of it! And many of the people I'd come into contact with who were using it or teaching it, I didn't think really understood it either. So if those who are doing it and teaching it can't come up with a coherent understanding of what it is and how you go about doing it, what hope have you got as a student?

Kitrina: So how did you start working differently?

David: Well, to recruit participants I had to spend time with them: that was the initial thing. But then you start to get to know people. It's really hard when you've been having a cup of tea with Ben and talking about his half-marathon, to then go away and read psychology or psychiatry books telling me what Ben *is* as *a person with schizophrenia*. I just felt, hang on a minute, what the research is saying doesn't fit my experience of this person. There was a real tension there. You see most of my life I have tended to put a lot of faith in received wisdom. When what I was taught didn't fit my life, I always thought it must be *me* that was wrong. As the years have gone by, having witnessed and experienced things that challenge what scientists have written, I've become more critical about 'accepted' knowledge and in recent years I've begun to realise why. But, practically, placed in context of my life, there was pressure to get my PhD finished – I'd already overrun, the funding had finished and I had to move out of my flat because the owners were selling. I needed to get the PhD done and find some work that paid. So, I went away with the transcripts and the task of 'writing up' my PhD. It was Harry Wolcott's work – that was probably the most important insight or teaching I had at that time – which showed me a far more human way of analysing, interpreting and writing research. Part of me still wanted neatness and resolution, answers, processes and methods, techniques to deal with the interview data, lots of it. But he taught me, through his writing, that it's OK to *engage* with the data, and *respond* to it according to what's in it, *not* rigidly follow pre-established techniques. I tried to do a thematic analysis, but I felt that was very superficial – themes didn't tell me anything about the nature of the participants' experiences. All I got from doing that type of analysis was a sequence of steps that people had been through in their initiation of physical activity. And I thought, God, there's a whole lot more in these interviews than that.

The work of storytellers

According to Smith and Sparkes (2009), a key strategic choice within narrative research is the question of how to explore and represent (for others) the stories that participants tell during interviews. We would like to consider two alternative approaches in this regard which we utilise in this book, at different times and for different purposes. To do so, we will reflect on the preceding interview which, in narrative terms, may be considered a co-constructed story about the experiences that led David to turn towards narrative research.

In presenting David's interview here as a storied account, we are working as *story-tellers*. From this perspective, analysis *is* the story, the story is already complete and is itself both theoretical and dialogical (Smith & Sparkes, 2009). That is, in the process of storying his experience, David was already utilising theory and analytic processes to interpret, form, shape and give meaning to his life experiences.

Narrative researchers who work as storytellers recognise that stories have intrinsic value in themselves. Through a storytelling approach it is possible to maintain the integrity of the story in order that others may *think with* the story from the perspective of their own life. Ellis and Bochner (2000, p. 753) characterise thinking with a story as 'allowing yourself to resonate with the story, reflect on it, become part of it'. For Frank (1995, p. 158), thinking with a story means 'joining with them, allowing one's own thoughts to adopt the story's immanent logic of causality, its temporality, and its narrative tensions . . . the goal is empathy, not as internalizing the feelings of the other, but as what Halpern calls "resonance with the other".'

Central to this process is the need for the reader to have access to a story that 'feels real' within the context of her or his (personal and/or professional) life experience. According to Frank (2000a), stories can be particularly effective in this regard because storytellers:

> offer those who do not share their form of life a glimpse of what it means to live informed by such values, meanings, relationships, and commitments. Others can witness what lives within the storyteller's community actually look, feel, and sound like. Storytellers tell stories because the texture of any form of life is so dense that no one can describe this form of life; the storyteller can only invite someone to come inside for the duration of the story. Those who accept an invitation into the storytelling relation open themselves to seeing (and feeling and hearing) life differently than they normally do. Listening is not so much a willing suspension of disbelief as a willing acceptance of different beliefs and of lives in which these beliefs make sense. Whether or how a story makes sense seems not so much an analytical question as an experiential one: Did the story draw others into its world far enough so that people's actions in that world seem reasonable in that world? Those who have accepted the invitation to the story may not choose to remain in the world of the story, but if the story works, then life in their worlds will seem different after they return there. (p. 361)

For Frank (2000a), therefore, social scientists have an ethical and intellectual obliga-tion to enter into storytelling relationships because stories communicate certain insights and 'truths' about people's lives which can be lost through taking a story apart. Our task as researchers is therefore – at times – to resist analysing others' stories; to, instead, 'step back from first-person testimony and allow those who testify to speak for themselves' (Frank, 2000a, p. 361). By presenting the interview above we have provided an example of how one individual (in this case David) authors and narrates his *own* life experiences. It is primarily David's voice we hear, without it being filtered through the analytic and interpretive interests of a researcher.

If one aim of social science research is to reduce the isolation many people experience in their lives and to bring about social justice and inclusion, then the storytelling approach has much to offer. To this end we, as researchers, bear an ethical obligation not only to be witnesses to such stories at the time of their creation (during the interview process), but also later through the way those stories are represented in research reports and publications. In adopting this approach we facilitate emergent ethics by circulating stories that need to be heard, by finding commonalities in those stories that we can share with others and by showing the, at times, 'inconvenient facts' that are hard to hear or that we might rather not consider (Frank, 2000a). To produce a story with this potential, a key task is to offer an evocative, emotionally revealing, empathetic portrayal of human experience with which the reader may 'connect' in some way. Arts-based approaches such as short stories, poetry, ethnodrama, film and music have great potential in this regard (see, for example, Angrosino, 1998; Chadwick, 2001b, 2006, 2007; Sparkes, 2002; Douglas & Carless, 2005, 2009b; Sparkes & Douglas, 2007; Carless & Sparkes, 2008; Carless & Douglas, 2009c). We utilise this kind of storytelling approach in chapters 2, 3, 10 and 11 of this book.

The work of story analysts

In contrast to storytellers, story analysts – described by some as those who conduct an *analysis of narratives* – *think about* a story which means 'to reduce it to content and then analyze that content' (Frank, 1995, p. 23). The story is thus broken down into themes or sub-categories that hold across stories or define particular threads of the story. According to Smith and Sparkes (2006, p. 185):

> Story analysts step outside or back from the story, employ analytical procedures, strategies or techniques in order to explore certain features of the story (e.g. content or structure) and carefully engage in abstract theorization about the story from a sociological, psychological and/or other disciplinary perspective.

There are numerous ways the preceding interview could be analysed and all relate to the purposes of the exploration and the audience to whom the findings will be revealed. The *types* of issues raised in David's story relating specifically to his journey towards narrative align with the accounts of other sport and exercise scholars who migrated to narrative partly as a consequence of their dissatisfaction with 'the way things are' in research terms (see Smith, 2010).

Another approach to analysing David' story might draw out the following points. The story is one where David's *experiences* of going into a particular place (hospital) brought back memories (of his family's trauma). These *feelings* (my dad might die) and awareness (this time is precious) sensitised him to some of the possible anxieties and issues in the lives of his potential participants and their families. These thoughts and feelings led to him *reflect* on and *question* his own motives (my questionnaire, my PhD) and ask himself – in light of these events in these people's lives – how important is *my* question. Because the story links past events with current and future events we, as listeners, can observe a narrative shift away from the *self* (what this individual wanted or needed) towards a focus and care directed at *others* (the person in the hospital bed who had just experienced a heart attack). As we follow the narrative flow, other events are brought in to show and explain how an original question about the effects of exercise on mood is reoriented to ask, for example: *How are people transformed through illness?* Taking a pedagogical orientation, the analysis might also explore a question such as: *How might personal transformation be addressed in the education and development of neophyte narrative researchers?*

Alongside these insights, we learn how embodied practicalities and societal expectations also influence the teller's ability to construct his story: the need to find paid employment, funding, pressure to complete a PhD. These practical limitations *also* shape the teller's story and choices. The story reveals how by reflecting on what he had learned led David to the conclusion that all the really important information 'went in the bin'. This was experienced as a tension between the academic requirements of doctoral study, and the possibilities and ethical imperatives of narrative research. These diverse analytic points illuminate how the questions *we* ask – as well as the theories and assumptions that underpin those questions – shape what we present as the 'findings' or 'results' of any analysis. We hope you will bear this point in mind as you consider the different story analyst approaches which we employ in chapters 4, 5, 6 and 9 of this book.

Both storyteller and story analyst approaches can form the basis of general knowledge through linking a particular case (or cases) with theory or with others' experience. For Ellis and Bochner (2000), lives are at the same time particular and general, since we are all embedded within cultural life as well as various social institutions. One way by which a story's generalisability can be realised therefore is when a reader experiences and understands another's life experiences or world through a *felt* sense of connection. By reflecting on how a particular individual's experiences 'fit' (or for that matter, challenge) personal experience (or existing theory), it is possible to create a more robust form of understanding which informs and translates to other comparable cases. Thus a reader gains insights into the worlds of other people (e.g. those diagnosed with a mental illness), and the workings of that world (e.g. the experiences of those who use mental health services).

We might point out that generalisations on the basis of a single case are routine in other areas of professional practice and policy. In courts of law, for example, precedents are sometimes set on the basis of one 'landmark' hearing. Here, future legal processes (applying to other similar cases) are informed by the outcome of a single previous case. In the aeronautical industry changes are made to designs, manufacturing and procedures on the basis of a single incident as documented by a 'black box' flight recorder. This might be an event that happened only once – such as an aeroplane crash – or it might even be an event that didn't happen at all – such as a 'near miss'. Here again, practice is informed or modified through reflecting on or theorising about a single case. These examples suggest to us that in the context of physical activity and mental health too, much can be learnt through in-depth study of the experiences of one or a few individuals.

A word on theory

We would like now to consider the theory that underpins our narrative approach to mental health research. In what follows, we outline:

(1) the social constructionist philosophy that underlies our work;
(2) the links between life stories, identity and mental health; and
(3) the ways personal stories are culturally shaped and influenced.

A social constructionist philosophy

We describe our research philosophy as a social constructionist perspective within the interpretive paradigm. Whereas the aims of research within the positivist paradigm are typically *explanation* and *control*, researchers who work under the assumptions of the interpretive paradigm are more interested in *understanding* and *illuminating* the nature of the social world and human experience (Sparkes, 1992). McLeod (1997) reminds us that social constructionist research takes as its goal the elucidation of *meaning* and, in so doing, often destabilises or calls into question existing assumptions regarding social experience. Thus, McLeod suggests, this kind of research meets one of the legitimate goals of systematic enquiry which is 'to sustain conversation and debate, rather than attempt to act as a "mirror to nature", as a source of foundational, universal truth' (p. 142).

Five key ideas underlie social constructionist approaches to research (developed from McLeod, 1997, p. 83) and characterise the research that informs this book. These are:

- a suspicion of taken-for-granted assumptions about the social world, which are understood as reinforcing the interests of powerful and dominant groups in society;
- a questioning or rejection of traditional positivist approaches to knowledge on the basis of their insufficient reflexivity;
- an appreciation that the goal of research and scholarship should not be to close down or finalise people's lives through producing knowledge that is claimed to be fixed and universally valid, but to open up an awareness of possibilities and horizons;
- the belief that the way we understand and make sense of the world is a result of historical and cultural processes of interaction and negotiation among different groups of people;
- a movement towards redefining psychological constructs such as 'mind', 'self', 'emotion' and 'mental health' as – in part at least – socially constructed as opposed to biologically determined processes.

Sparkes and Smith (2008) describe narrative inquiry as one dimension of a constructionist paradigm which offers the epistemological opportunity to be both a way of *telling* about our lives as well as a method or means of *knowing* about lives (see also Etherington, 2003, 2007b; Holstein & Gubrium, 2005). Several prominent narrative theorists (e.g. Bruner, 1986; McAdams, 1993; Brooks, 1994; McLeod, 1997; Crossley, 2000) have articulated the view that, as humans, we are fundamentally storied beings and that our experiences are closely intertwined with the stories we and others tell of our lives. From this perspective, a two-way relationship can be seen where our stories both *shape* and are *shaped by* our embodied experiences (see Carless, in press). Narrative inquiry is therefore well suited to understanding individuals within their social contexts, as active agents in the creation of identities and selves, yet at the same time shaped and constrained by cultural expectations, roles and relationships. For this reason, stories shared by individuals tell us not only about their lives and experiences, but also about the society and culture in which they are embedded.

Life stories and mental health

There are good reasons to believe that the experience of mental health and illness is related to a person's ability and opportunity to create and share stories of their life. According to Dan McAdams (1993), developing one's life story contributes to mental health and well-being through bringing a sense of meaning and purpose to life which helps avoid malaise and stagnation. A critical link between life stories and mental health seems to be the need to establish and maintain a coherent identity which brings a sense of meaning and purpose to our lives. A sense of identity, in Norman Denzin's (2003, p. 91) terms, is 'a way of knowing that no matter where I put myself that I am not necessarily what's around me' which helps preserve a degree of stability and continuity across changing life events, circumstances and contexts. By linking our past, present and future through a life story, a coherent identity can be developed which 'makes sense' across disparate experiences. The maintenance of a sense of coherence, Clive Baldwin (2005, p. 1023) suggests, 'is an overarching feature of a life-project and productive of well-being and (arguably) its loss is a feature of mental ill-health such as in schizophrenia or post-traumatic stress disorder'.

Meaning and coherence are not, however, a 'given' – these qualities are by no means inherent features of either experience or stories. Some experiences appear meaningless and some stories may seem incoherent. Instead, research has shown that meaning and coherence are created through creating and telling stories of one's experience (see Smith & Sparkes, 2002). In other words, people 'achieve' or 'realise' meaning and coherence by successfully engaging in the task of storying their experience. This finding is significant in that it begs the question: if we require storytelling opportunities to bring meaning and coherence to our life, what happens when storytelling opportunities are denied?

This question is a concern for us because the experience of mental illness (particularly in its more severe forms) can deny a person both the ability and the opportunity to author their own life story. According to Baldwin (2005), cognitive difficulties or the loss of language can result in individuals losing the ability to construct and articulate a coherent life story. At the same time, an 'individual's interactions with others may be restricted by a condition that results in decreased opportunities to launch and maintain narratives' (Baldwin, 2005, p. 1023). In this regard, problems with thought processes, communication, social connectedness and/or activity can together conspire to deny a person with mental health problems the opportunity to both create and share stories of her or his life. A likely consequence of this denial is that the individual will be limited or restricted in terms of the avenues through which she may develop and maintain a coherent, meaningful identity.

Cultural stories and mental health

It is significant that, while stories are personal, they are at the same time shaped by cultural factors. That is, our own life story is shaped and constrained by more general narrative scripts and plots that circulate within our particular culture. It is very difficult (if not impossible) to tell a story of one's life *without* in some way being influenced by a more broadly understood narrative. 'Going to school', 'getting a job' and 'getting fit' are examples of stories that are generally circulated in our culture as necessary and (to some extent) desirable. They are stories we are expected to cultivate. Stories which transgress these expectations – such as stories which tell of 'not going to school', 'not getting a job', or 'not getting fit' – can sometimes be difficult to 'hear' or accept because they contravene the expected story. These alternative stories, while not inherently good or bad in themselves, present an atypical plot with a lack of shared cultural conventions and reference points.

In illness contexts, Frank (1995) shows how a dominant medical narrative – the restitution narrative – acts to shape and constrain individual stories (and experiences) of illness. This type of narrative, Frank (1995, p. 77) suggests, is 'filled out with talk of tests and their interpretation, treatments and their possible outcomes, the competence of physicians, and alternative treatments'. The basic plot of the restitution narrative is 'yesterday I was healthy, today I'm sick, but tomorrow I'll be healthy again'. While this plot may 'fit' some people's illness experiences, it is unlikely to be helpful in the context of more severe forms of mental illness when restitution (i.e. a return to previous health as it once was) may be unrealistic or even impossible. For people in this situation, the assumption of restitution ('cure') is problematic – or even hopeless – because a future free of illness simply cannot be envisaged. Striving to 'get back' to something that is elusive or impossible risks leading to hopelessness and without hope it becomes impossible to find reasons to carry on.

The power of the medical narrative to influence the life story of people with mental illness is recognised by Baldwin (2005) when he suggests that the experiences accompanying serious mental health problems threaten narrative agency. At these times, the 'big story' of mental illness disrupts individuals' ability and opportunity to maintain or create a personal story which fits their life experiences. This narrative damage is in itself a further threat to mental health which can compromise identity development and well-being (Lysaker & Lysaker, 2002, 2006). If a loss of narrative agency and continuity is to be prevented, Baldwin (2005) suggests, it is necessary to challenge disruptive and limiting illness narratives through the creation and realisation of counter stories that are individual, enabling and meaningful.

A word on method

Our focus in this book is on understanding how physical activity and sport can contribute to recovery in the context of mental illness. A key focus in exploring this question is the meaning that involvement in physical activity and sport holds in the lives of people who have experienced mental health problems. As we have already discussed, this focus necessitates studying the experiences of individuals, which we have done primarily through gathering and exploring their stories.

Participants in the research

The foundation of our understanding about the potential of physical activity and sport has come from data gathered through interviews conducted over an 8-year period with 13 men and women aged between 24 and 43. All these individuals had been diagnosed with a severe and enduring mental illness (such as schizophrenia or bipolar disorder) and all were involved in some kind of sport or physical activity. We invited individuals to take part in the research on the basis of: (i) their personal experience of both serious mental illness and sport/exercise participation; (ii) their willingness to take part in the research; and (iii) mental health professionals' assessment that the individual was sufficiently 'well' to participate. The research was granted ethical clearance by the local National Health Service Trust, participation was on a voluntary basis and all those who agreed to take part provided informed consent. The research began as part of David's PhD studies (Carless, 2003) and has subsequently been developed and published in a variety of international peer-reviewed journals (Carless, 2007, 2008; Carless & Douglas, 2004, 2008a, 2008b, 2008c, 2008d, 2009c; Carless & Sparkes, 2008).

Added to this – and alongside the above research – we have also learned a great deal about mental health, identity development and psychological well-being, through our research with elite sportspeople (Douglas, 2004, 2009; Douglas & Carless, 2006, 2008a, 2008b, 2008c, 2008d, 2009a, 2009b; Carless & Douglas, 2009a). This work draws on data gathered through interviews conducted over a 6-year period with nine female professional golfers. Since we completed our doctoral studies we have conducted several other research projects and evaluations (e.g. Douglas & Carless, 2005; Women's Sports Foundation, 2005) and the insights gained in these projects have also contributed to how we have conducted, analysed, interpreted and presented what we have learnt.

We have also presented our research to participants, other service users and their families, friends, academic peers, practitioners, health professionals, students and other interested people. In a sense, these individuals have also been 'participants' in our research because these interactions have extended our learning and deepened our understanding. We have also continued to interview people whose life experiences extend – sometimes complexify and deepen – the knowledge we share. For example, in chapter 10, we present interviews with three practitioners who deliver physical activity programmes in mental health contexts. We invited these practitioners to share their experiences as part of our aim to 'complete the circle' and point towards future sport provision and practice within mental health contexts.

Collecting stories

Our approach to collecting individual's stories – our research 'data' – has been to (where possible) use a life history approach to interviewing which begins with what Wolcott (1994) terms the *grand tour* question: 'Tell me about your life.' That is, we asked participants to describe their life, in their own words, from childhood to the present day. Doing so, we feel, respects the individual, their personal journey, their way of describing their life and the details that are meaningful to them. Along this narrative journey, we asked the individual to tell us about his or her experience of physical activity, sport and mental health. Throughout the interviews, we tried to respond to the stories which were shared – sometimes by offering stories of our own experience and sometimes by asking further questions such as: 'What did that mean to you?' 'Why did you do that?' 'How did that make you feel?' As such, the stories we collected are a reconstruction of the individual's experience, told at a specific time, to a specific person for a specific aim. We recognise therefore, that all the stories were shaped, to an extent, by our own interests and ways of thinking.

We have been aware of some potential risks in taking this research approach, particularly in the context of serious mental illness. By interviewing participants we have invited them to tell their own stories yet, as Brendan Stone (2004) observes, therein lays a risk. In his words:

> to formulate a narrative will necessitate a willed passage into and through the same spaces of self – thought, memory and emotion – in which the illness has been, and possibly still is, manifest … All of this, I want to suggest, means the narrative journey may be a perilous one. (p. 20)

Our desire to minimise the perils of the 'narrative journey' – the dangers arising from talking about and revisiting potentially traumatic life phases – led us to draw on other forms of data collection to reduce the possible demands placed on the participants through taking part in multiple interviews, focus groups and feedback sessions. In some cases, it also meant that we refrained from sharing our interpretations with some participants as a result of an expressed wish to *not* revisit the interview once it was complete.

To minimise these risks we utilised the techniques and principles of ethnography. Initially, over a period of 18 months David participated in day-to-day life at a vocational rehabilitation day centre for people with serious mental illness, taking part in sport and exercise groups as well as social activities. This period of immersion 'in the field' supported the development of a degree of trust, rapport and familiarity. At the time we were also beginning to be aware that, from an ethical point of view, there is much we can bring to the lives of those we conduct research with, as well as what we take from them. *What* or *who* an individual becomes is shaped, in part, by the body-self path they choose. For Frank, those with a dyadic body 'exist for each other: They exist for the task of discovering what it means to live for other bodies' (1995, p. 37).

Musing on this issue we wondered if we could use our knowledge and skills in sport to provide an activity that wasn't currently included at this particular day centre. After tentatively discussing the idea with staff, their enthusiastic response led us to gain external funding to start a golf group. As Kitrina is a qualified golf coach, she also attended the centre on a weekly basis and coached the golf activity group. Our actions therefore transgressed many barriers normally established between participants and researchers as we became actively involved in practice and provision. Reflecting on these choices it appears to us now that in this regard we were developing a type of action research – collecting data, learning, teaching and developing sport strategies and testing and refining them alongside the original research questions we were exploring. We believe this is one of the strengths of the narrative constructionist paradigm, in that it allows our researcher-selves to develop and explore opportunities that arise within the course of our research as we ourselves become more aware.

The above actions meant we utilised a variety of data collection methods in addition to life story interviews. These were:

- *Informal interviews and observations.* This included conversations and general interaction with mental health professionals and coaching personnel during sport and exercise activities and day-to-day life at a mental health vocational rehabilitation day centre.
- *Formal interviews and focus groups with mental health professionals.* We also conducted interviews and focus groups with the lead clinical psychologist at the day centre, the lead physiotherapist, an occupational manager, an exercise leader, an activity co-ordinator, a dance and movement specialist and several care workers who worked closely with individual participants. These interviews were recorded and transcribed verbatim.
- *Analysis of medical records.* Given the diverse issues that may influence mental health and illness across the lifespan, we felt that – with four participants – additional understanding might be gained through considering the individual's medical history. The ethics committee gave us permission to access medical records to gain information on course of illness and treatment history. While these records are in themselves a situated (medical) narrative, they provided us with some sense of the chronology of medical history which allowed us to be more aware of potentially sensitive issues.

Exploring and representing stories

The 'data' that accumulated through the processes we describe above is amenable to a variety of analytic approaches. All these approaches may be considered alternative ways to explore and represent the participants' stories – each with particular strengths and weaknesses and, therefore, suited to different purposes. In an effort to glean as much as we can from participants' stories, we have utilised a variety of different analytic procedures, often through a multi-stage process. This process has been a form of ongoing analysis because we often think about our experiences even when we are not 'at work' – perhaps when out running, walking or surfing, or when playing or listening to music. Paradigm shifts in our understanding of the 'data' have occurred during all these times.

Our analytic approaches may be divided according to the *storyteller* and *story analyst* approaches we described earlier in this chapter. Both begin with close and repeated readings of the interview transcripts, field notes or other written records. Through this process we aim to become 'immersed in the data'. When using a storytelling approach, we try to remain in the story, perhaps making notes or margin comments, attending to our own feelings as we read through the text. We then share these thoughts and feelings with each other and discuss what we each learned from the story. Having a 'critical friend' or 'outsider' has proved a supportive structure – we both find it adds not only rigour to the research, but also brings a shared sense of purpose and enjoyment to what can be a solitary and lonely task. The usually necessary step of reducing the story to a publishable length follows our discussions as one of us begins reducing and cutting segments which are not essential to the story plot, which are overly repetitive or for which there is too much detail.

In the case of a story analyst approach, we begin with a content analysis to identify and code themes arising from the data using quotations as the unit of analysis (see Sparkes, 2005). From here, a variety of analytical strategies are possible (see Lieblich *et al.*, 1998; Riessman, 2008). One we have used in this book (chapters 4 and 5) is described by Sparkes (2005) as *an analysis of structure and form*. This approach to analysis is important, we think, because aspects of structure – as much as the literal content of a story – express the identity, perceptions and values of the storyteller (Sparkes, 2005). Our aim through this type of analysis is to communicate (through linking the stories with culturally available narratives) an understanding of the meaning and value of physical activity and sport within the context of participants' life experiences.

Key points

- In this chapter we have considered both the theory and practice of narrative research in an effort to bring a level of transparency to our research. Through reproducing an interview Kitrina conducted with David regarding his own journey towards narrative we provide an example of how research is an ongoing, evolving process that necessarily affects the researcher/s, the participants and ultimately the 'findings' that are produced. In so doing, we have offered our rationale for narrative inquiry and shown how using narrative theory can illuminate our own lives and ethical choices, as well as providing a lens through which to understand the lives of our participants.
- We choose to reveal ourselves and our own experiences in this chapter not because we think researchers' lives are particularly important, but rather as an ethical act of *standing with* those we research. By stepping out of the shadows of traditional scientific writing, we strive for a degree of reflexivity through which we reveal ourselves – to participants and readers alike – as vulnerable human beings who also struggle with the tensions inherent in life and work.
- We have described two alternative approaches to working with stories – that of *storyteller* and *story analyst* – and provided details of and rationales for our use of these approaches in the chapters which follow.
- We have presented narrative inquiry as particularly suited to understanding individuals within their social contexts, as active agents in the creation of identities and selves, yet at the same time shaped and constrained by cultural expectations roles, and relationships. For this reason, stories shared by individuals tell us not only about their lives and what is meaningful for them, but also about the society and culture in which they are embedded.

Part II

Understanding physical activity and sport in mental health

Personal stories of sport, physical activity and mental health

If you want to know me, then you must know my story, for my story defines who I am. And if I want to know myself, to gain insight into the meaning of my own life, then I, too, must come to know my own story.

Dan McAdams (1993, p. 11)

In this chapter, we begin to consider the relationship between physical activity, sport and mental health through a *storyteller* approach. To do so, we present life stories of two individuals, Laura and Colin, who kindly agreed to be interviewed during the course of our research.

As we discussed in chapter 2, by taking a storyteller approach we foreground a 'complete' story and resist 'taking the story apart' through analytic procedures or techniques. We do this in the recognition that stories fulfil a necessary and important role in human and social science by providing insights and understandings that cannot be gained through other means of communication (such as scientific reports or analyses). McLeod (1997) observes that:

> One of the distinctive features of the modern world … has been the tendency to ignore and diminish the significance of stories. We can easily recognise the entertainment value of stories, but we do not take them *seriously* … The growth of science and technology over the last 200 years has been associated with a gradual loss of legitimacy of stories as a way of communicating truths about the world, to be replaced by a belief in the validity of scientific procedures as a means of arriving at reliable and accurate knowledge. (p. 29)

Through failing to take stories seriously, we are concerned that certain ways of knowing – about the world, about people's lives, about experience – risk being lost. One such loss might be a sense of *context*; another might be an understanding of *connections.* Stories can remind us of potentially significant contextual factors which can be lost through scientific methods, while making connections between disparate and apparently unrelated events to help us develop a rich understanding of a person's life and experiences. Rita Charon (2006, p. 194) observes how 'The moral and aesthetic resonances of novels, poems, and plays offer different kinds of evidence from that offered by scientific experiments, and yet it is an evidence that counts very much in understanding human's predicaments.' In a similar vein, Chadwick (2009, p. 22) suggests that life is bigger than reason and, therefore, that at times 'the melody of behaviour, is better captured in art, by the kinematic representation of a play or a novel than by using the static mode of the binoculars of a questionnaire'.

The stories which follow were developed from the transcripts of life history interviews with Laura and Colin. We recognise three aesthetic processes which were at work during the task of shaping and crafting these stories for representation here:

- *Selection.* Given the focus of this book on physical activity and sport for mental health, we have selectively focused on moments and sections of each person's story which we felt were more closely related to this topic. Thus the stories which follow should not be considered 'the' story of Laura or Colin's life, but rather 'a' story of her/his life.
- *Editing.* The stories as told during the interviews were simply too long to be published in their entirety. Through an editing process we tried to distil the essence of each individual's story in a way that would, hopefully, remain faithful to the original life story while being interesting and engaging for readers.
- *Reorganising.* Stories told in an oral and conversational form (e.g. during an interview) do not necessarily 'work' effectively when reproduced verbatim in written form. In recognition of this, we sometimes reorganised the order or flow of the original narratives in an effort to improve continuity, coherence, intelligibility, aesthetic form and/or impact.

Throughout these processes, we worked to retain a feel for how Laura and Colin told their own stories to us during the interviews. Important for us in this regard was to retain (for example) idiosyncrasies of speech, unusual expressions, descriptive details and personal reflections. To this end, the stories which follow are presented in the individual storyteller's own words as spoken during our interviews. For reasons of confidentiality, specific details (such as names, places and dates) have, where necessary, been changed.

Laura's story

I can remember my primary school vividly, you were allowed to work at your own pace and I loved it. There was no traditional hockey or cricket, we just played games and it was fun. At home, perhaps because I'm an only child, I was encouraged to do something if I wanted to do it. So, I started ballet classes when I was three, and tap, and I also started swimming. Now apparently, at swimming, I was a bit of a demon! My swimming teacher was lovely, but he did threaten to throw you in at the deep end if you didn't behave! I remember swimming from being older, when it was fun, but my parents say when I was very little I used to spend the whole time screaming and clinging to my swimming teacher. Neither mum nor dad could swim well so I probably inherited their nervousness, but once I got going I did all my swimming badges. I can remember being appalled that I had to wear a swimming hat for Galas, and I hated the damn thing, but I did love swimming and swam twice a week.

Having started ballet at three, I took to dancing like a duck to water, and apparently I had the odd tantrum there as well. I think most of my self-expression, extremes of mood, which have become more obvious now I'm bipolar – I'm very much, 'you get what you see' – were clearly apparent when I was tiny as well. By the time I was eleven I was dancing every day with one day off on a Sunday. I actually went to audition for a place at the Royal Ballet School. Fortunately I didn't get in, I mean look at me – short, dumpy ballerinas with big boobs don't get much money do they? But I carried on at that level and intensity 'til I went to secondary school.

That was a bit of a shock to the system. I was offered a full scholarship, but I really wanted to go to that school because of the lemon curd sandwiches at the interview. Boarding school at eleven was fantastic and horrific in equal quantities. It teaches you self-reliance, but takes away any sense of normal relationships. I was still doing dancing but just twice a week, but we had games teachers who were bullies and who would only take the ones who really shone, and would only work with them. I liked hockey, probably because I didn't get shouted at, which is an awful thing to say, but I was really tiny, and I think I was probably a bit too weak and weedy, and we had that awful thing about communal showers. You wonder where the people who run schools or those who make policies grew up, 'cause every pubescent child hates showers!

When I was in the lower sixth I fell and shattered the cartilage on my left knee, so I left school with quite a bad knee and went to university. From the point of view of work, the degree was great, but from having time for anything else, it became more and more difficult, and I couldn't dance because I damaged my knee, and there was no swimming pool. So the two things I really enjoyed and was good at, I was grounded. Uni sport was also very competitive, the sort of atmosphere where you weren't encouraged unless you were good enough to play for the BUSA team. So I don't think I did any formal exercise. I did go in the sports hall – to take exams!

If I went home though, I'd do lots of adventure things – canoeing, climbing, caving – and I loved it. You're part of a team, there was no competition, but you were encouraged to check the person behind and in front, I enjoyed that. There was a big group of us, all ages, and we achieved things and I used to letterbox on Dartmoor and I got my 100 club membership and I was really proud of that.

I first got ill when I was sixteen, depression was the problem. Everyone thought, 'Wow, that's a girl who's going places,' yet actually, I was profoundly depressed. I used to spend hours crying but it wasn't really diagnosed, and nothing really happened. It settled when I first went to university, but when it flared up in the fourth year, I think 'cause I was in a much bigger environment and much less secure, I started to become much more brittle and I got very depressed very quickly and I was hospitalised. I think I was aware that something wasn't quite right, and I went to the student health centre and it all gets a bit blurry then, I'm not sure who was involved and I had a few really quite bad episodes. One which required hospitalisation, and it was absolutely horrendous. It was in one of the old-style hospitals, you know, that had its own farm and train line, yeah … it's the only time I've been offered hard drugs. The first two days I was there I didn't eat because nobody told me how to get food, and when we went to get something we had to register and I was number 14, I still have a dislike of the number 14, and they would use a number instead of your name, it was very dehumanising.

Then I got better and the general practice department helped me organise an elective at a medical museum which I loved, and I caught up and graduated on time. I think if you are vulnerable you actually make a better doctor, you can understand what people mean when they say, 'this is awful,' and so I finished medical school and knew I was a good doctor, basically, because I spent time with people and because of my own problems I could listen in a way that would help them.

By then I was aware that I was vulnerable, so I applied for house jobs nearer home and the first one was surgical. I enjoyed that, but I was never cut out to be a surgeon, you know, there was a danger that someone's appendectomy scar would have flowers and beads attached to it. I had a little wobble in the middle of that job. That was the first time I became aware that night shifts were going to be a problem. But I finished my six months' surgery and I got really, really lovely reports, and I was really pleased and they were pleased with me. Then I went to North Devon to do medicine – that is a fantastic hospital. I did endocrinology, general medical take, and oncology, and I was really well all the way through. There was none of this, 'I'm a doctor, you're a physio or nurse', we'd all go out together. You're made to feel valued for what you do but you have a respect for everyone. I like to look back at my reports, 'cause it shows I was good at my job. Then my next job was paediatrics, and it was a small hospital and I really flourished, and I knew I was going to be there for at least a year, so I actually joined the gym, and used the pool.

But then I moved to the children's hospital. This is my horror story. This is where it all falls apart because the children's hospital is big, and I think the biggest problem was I didn't make friends, and I know that sounds primary school-ish, when I got there they messed up my accommodation, and it kind of disintegrated from there. The environment was 'career paediatricians' and I felt I was expected to be like that. So I actually went to the GP fairly soon, and I know exactly when it happened because I was walking to my doctor's appointment, and somebody came out from the pub, just a random bloke, grabbed me and said, 'Look at this! This is world news! You've got to see this, it's awful!' And I saw the plane go in to the twin towers on the television, which wasn't relevant (even though it was horrific), but it fixed it in time for me. That's my kind of 'D-day', that's where things really unravelled very quickly, and I became really profoundly suicidal. I ended up going to day hospital, and plummeted into the middle of the psych services. It's weird, because I can remember everything up to that point chronologically very clearly, but from there, there is a big chunk, probably, three or four years, that are just a blur of this happening and that happening, and a nasty blur as well. The psych services can be a very cruel place, you get all sorts of labels about being manipulative, and about having personality disorders, and actually you are just struggling with a problem, you are awash with bizarre medication, and you've lost any form of normality in your life, any regularity that you might have, and your life is falling completely to bits, and then they are judging you from there. Rather than saying, well this is Laura, and this is what has happened to her. I wouldn't wish it on anyone, those first few years.

The day centre I went to originally had an exercise group that used the little gym, and a physio came in and did circuits for very poorly people, and because she had knowledge of sport and of mental health, she didn't do anything too hard, but she could get you into doing little bits and bobs, so I went to that, and I did gardening and pottery, and art. Then I joined in the walking group which was run by a chap who my headmaster would call 'a man who walks with purpose,' and he managed to get this raggle-taggle group into a brisk walk across the Downs, and we'd come back and have lunch and people would chat and then go back to your life. That was a really good example of how outpatient care was run then, you get a good square meal and you are safe.

Then I got discharged and you go from this very supportive atmosphere to *nothing* – there is no middle ground. For several years I was bouncing backwards and forwards between the GP's and the psychiatrist, who wouldn't give me a diagnosis. There is a trend towards that at the moment, not labelling people, calling them clients. *This is not a life choice it's an illness!* So my GP at the time agreed that we were in a stagnant position, and so she sent me for a second opinion. They said, 'Well look – you are bipolar, you have clearly been bipolar since adolescence and we should recognise that. You clearly have a long-term problem, you are never going to get rid of this.' Which, again, was important to hear: because I have a diagnosis it's almost as if people can respect the diagnosis but they can't respect the disordered person. So now I have a *reason* that's acceptable to health professionals, it's acceptable to the general public, and that means I can access the right type of medication and the right types of support. I have a very strict regulated life and I live within limits that I know I can control.

So I got bounced back again to the psych services. In the interim the day care centre had changed, they still had a few classes but little camaraderie, and to me it felt like 'them and us'. It was 'we are going to prescribe you art' instead of 'why don't you come and do art?' It wasn't really a huge success because they weren't really offering any support and so I drifted really, which put my partner, who is stuck with being my carer, under huge strain, and it was all a bit of a mess.

Then we moved house and that meant a different GP and day centre. He's excellent, he treats me with professional courtesy, he has a laugh with me and will tease me, but he's been really good at picking up on triggers. He read my details and his approach is 'Yes this is bipolar, let's manage it.' The crisis team then referred me to the occupational health team and although they are the new breed of day hospital, they seem to focus on getting you some sort of outcome. My key worker's view was 'yes, you have these problems, but how can we address them?' She suggested doing some physical activity groups, which was something I would be able to carry on after I've been discharged. I had quite a long period of no physical activity basically because there was nothing on offer, then, about two years ago, I got the opportunity to go to a badminton group. I think I would have struggled if I had been very poorly: people think, 'Oh! It's just a badminton session,' but it's not, there's a hell of a lot more to deal with. It's like, if you got your computer out and ran like, fourteen web searches, and eight lots of Photoshop and Word for Windows, it would gradually crank to a halt, and that's exactly what going to the gym is like for me. It's like, putting myself in a position of vulnerability, having to meet lots of new people and things that aren't necessarily predictable. I can't always say who's going to be there, or who's not going to be there, and that's aside to any other symptoms I have. Yeah, it's quite a big thing.

But what playing badminton has done, from a physical activity point of view is, it's been the finger that's pushed the dominoes. 'Cause after I started to play badminton, one of my best friends said 'You're getting fit, hmmm, I'm getting lardy. What are we going to do about it?' So doing the badminton in a mental health setting gave me the confidence to start aerobics at the local sport centre with a friend and possibly because the badminton group isn't just mental health professionals – you are interacting with coaches as well – it gave me confidence to go up to the teacher and say 'This is my problem, I'm bipolar, sometimes it might be a bit much for me, sometimes I might not grasp things if I'm not feeling very well, so could you just keep a vague eye and point me in the right direction.' And that was very successful so then we ended up going to body pump as well.

I definitely get a buzz afterwards, I feel like I have achieved something and I feel, well, energised. I definitely feel very good that I can join something 'normal'. The teacher is very dedicated, but not draconian, so much so that on a few occasions, when the others haven't been able to go, I've gone on my own. I'm sure I wouldn't have done that if I hadn't done the badminton group.

And now things are even more unusual because I am mad *and* pregnant. We did try aqua natal, but the slight problem is – not from a pregnancy point of view but from a mental health point of view – because the class starts at 10 o'clock in the morning, it's too early. One of the ways I manage my bipolar is to have a very strict routine, and a lot of psychotropic medication does have sedative properties, so you take it at night, so it does take a little time to get up and running in the morning.

After the baby is born I will be discharged, so I'm not sure if I will have access to the physical activity run by the trust. The badminton group they run is less threatening than a normal class. There's a little group of us that stay for a drink in the café, and we play together, we've built up a nice social group as well, but three of them have been approached about attending a move-on class so I'm likely to lose my friends. The big advantage of that group is because nobody expects anything of you, you can go even if you are not feeling that great, it's easy, whereas, if you are not feeling so good, and you are attending a mainstream group, it's much easier *not* to go, 'cause you feel you might not cope. The other thing, the badminton was stoking all the other exercise and I don't think I could regularly do a class by myself at the local gym.

The psych services give you something to pin your activities on, and when you are not feeling great, and you do something that's easy access, you can do it, and because it makes you feel better it makes it possible for you to do that bit more. When you are discharged, you lose that. It does have an important role in that the supported stuff makes 'normal' things easier to access, so without the security of supported activities, community sport becomes more of a mountain to climb. The psych services are weird, 'cause they build you up for discharge, which is great, because you probably don't need to see the psychiatrist regularly if you are stable, but it also curtails your access to all those things that help you stay stable.

From when you start to get poorly, to when you accept the diagnosis, you are putting your brain in society's straitjacket – that expects you to conform in a certain way. When you can relax and accept who you are and the problems, challenges or bonuses it might give you, you can blossom in a different way. It might be very different to the expected careers path! It's a better way – it suits me much better anyway. People assume with bipolar that you don't want it, but actually, if you took me back ten years, when I was a really high-flying achiever – the state that everyone assumes that I want to get back to – very few people bother to check in and find out that now I am happier than I have ever been and I am probably well-er than I have ever been. Now I accept my own limits and diagnosis – and use it.

Colin's story

I think I was talented. I think that's what it was. I played for the school when I was young – eleven, twelve or thirteen. I played for the juniors, made two appearances, but scored one goal and I always remember that. I remember going down the wing, 'cause I played left half, and this ball came over from one of the players and I just looked up and hit it and it went behind the goalkeeper's head! I just took it as normal, just hit the ball and it just went in. It was great! I felt really, you know, just felt great. Thought I'd achieved something. We were at home against our local rivals, Bridgeside, who used to play at Borough Park. I knew the goalkeeper you see, he played for City in the end, Peter Reeves. I can't remember what the score was but that was our local rivalry. That was when I first started really. But I used to play football, outside, in the house gardens on my own, just kicking a ball. So really I started when I was about seven or eight I suppose. I used to play football over the park, Sunday mornings with my friends and then Sunday afternoons again, another match. I just got addicted to it. It just went from there really.

When I was about twenty I started playing in the local league for Wanderers. That was my first football team, I played for other teams, but I think that was my favourite one 'cause I was there the longest – about four or five years. I used to play left back. We had an injury to one of our players, Terry Stone, he played left back and I took his place. And then what happened, the manager, Steve Corr, was in goal and he had a knee injury and I took over in goal. I made about 100 appearances in goal for the team.

I used to train over the park on my own. There's one of my favourite photos, one of the earlier ones before I had my breakdown. That's the house in the background and Woodland Park where I used to train on my own – skills, like. I used to kick the ball in the air, let it bounce, catch it, do shooting practice with two footballs. I used to ride a bike at the time, and I did a bit of swimming then, so I was quite fit really. And football just gave me a kick, you know, enthusiasm! I just thought it was a great game, it really gave me a lift. I've always loved the game.

I stopped football when I was unwell 'cause I was pretty low. That was my first breakdown then. I was twenty-eight, I can remember that very well. I think it was anxiety, stress, work, everything, like. I'd just done too much and it hit me for six. I just had a breakdown and that was it really. I was over at my mother's house, I used to go to sleep a lot, I switched off. I used to go into my own little synchronisation sort of thing, I used to sleep for hours and hours. The head doctor of the mental side of the hospital came round to the house and saw me a couple of times; come to my room, just say 'we're checking you out', ask me a few questions. She knew I was very low and she said you've gotta go to Brentree – we're taking you in.

So I was at Brentree Hospital for a bit, about two or three months I think it was. I was so bored in there – nothing to do. I just stayed in the ward and just went to bed and that was it. I'd just get up, have something to eat, a cup of tea, sit in the television room, talk to somebody and then just hang about for a couple of hours unless a doctor wanted to see me. I think that's what made me go to sleep 'cause I was bored, depressed. I thought, well, I've got nothing else to do. I just want to go to sleep. The doctors knew that as well, my morale was still quite low, that's why they asked me to do some activities. They tried to get me to do exercise just to get me out of that system.

It was the group, starting to talk to people, and the medication I think. I started taking medication and saw a few doctors and I started getting better. The medication helped me to stabilise myself. I started talking and got out of my shell. It was important to talk to people, communicate with people and once I started talking to people it gave me more confidence. So all that was on my own part really, I did it myself, started to talk to people myself.

I started with some activities like going somewhere in the van for a couple of hours. Chaps would come round and take us out, so that was like a walking group really, just to get out of the hospital. And then I started going to gym and went to OT and then I started going swimming – that was it then. It wasn't so bad then. My confidence came back. I was actually on the road to recovery.

Once I got in the gym I used to go and do those exercises on the bars, the weightlifting, and the bike and what have you. I was doing it every day, five days I think, about nine o'clock in the morning. It was an early session! It was hard work 'cause I wasn't so strong then but I was there about forty-five minutes. 'Cause I was doing exercises I felt a bit better like, felt more, a bit of energy, felt a bit stronger. Rather than feeling low, when I was doing some activity – the exercises – I felt better. I gained something out of it. 'Cause when I was low I had different mood levels – the medication I was on that'd alternate the moods I was in. When I took that it gave me a lift. But when I was doing exercises it was similar to that, it gave me a lift similar to the medication 'cause I'd done something, I'd participated in something. It was something out of the blue that came to me and I just had a go. I just attacked it in a normal way and, you know, I appreciated what I'd done in the end. I got something out of it.

It was only a couple of weeks. After that I knew I'd had enough of it – that was enough of the gym for me I think. It did enough to boost my morale. I was a little bit better then and I could do other things like routine work, therapy work, go to OT, play table tennis, do quizzes and I used to do a bit of cooking there as well. I used to make my own way down to the OT, whereas sometimes when I was low they used to come over and meet me to make sure I would turn up. That's the time they knew I was low – depressed.

It could have been a year, or, I think it was, yeah. It took quite a long time to get back to normal, the person as I was. 'Cause I made a recovery and then I started playing football again, just kind of natural really. I've just always been mad on sports! The sort of games that I played in the past, when I was younger, I sort of started back playing them again. It's just the enthusiasm really, that's what has changed my life. Well, apart from the music I would say. If I didn't play football or have any music I don't think I'd be here today. I think it's kept me going. Well, it brings all your talent out, your ability in other words. It brings the, say, the cleverness out of you. 'Cause we've all got talents, everybody's got some talents, doesn't matter if it's art or it's football, engineering, cars, anything, I think we've all got a talent. Mine is activity – sports. Keeps me going, keeps the adrenalin going.

I like to play other games – it's just, like, *doing*. When you do all these other sports it's not so boring. I think it's better for a person to do a different sport, see how you get on, rather than just sticking to the one game. Skittles, I played that for must be sixteen years now I think I've been with the team! I've been with the team so long it's like a family really. Pool, I play pool sometimes – that's the other sport. But it's mostly the football and walking really. It's basically football, swimming – a bit of swimming – walking with the walking group and badminton sometimes.

I feel more relaxed after I've been swimming – something about the water makes you feel good. When I was young I was afraid of the water. My mum used to encourage me to jump into the water and I was just terrified of water! But I met a chap that used to live over near Oakside Baths where I used to go that taught me how to swim – breaststroke and front crawl – and gave me a lot of confidence in the water. I still get the same confidence 'cause I know that I can swim. It's like when I go on holiday, I know that I can swim in the sea, I'm quite a strong swimmer, I know that I can do it – it gives me a buzz.

I would say the last time I swam was about a month ago with Simon. I was looking forward to it 'cause I know it'll just come natural, see. Switch off and concentrate on swimming a few lengths, just taking it steady. Think about other things as well, what's happening and that. It could be what you saw the other day, or what you're gonna do an hour after you've finished swimming, or your mother and father. Depends what mood you're in. If you're in a sad mood you might think of your dad, I would anyway, always think of my dad now and again. Get flashes with him like, but I think it's a good thing in a way. 'Cause I was so close with him – when I went to our dad's funeral I was in hell of a state. I cried my eyes out. Terrible. Nobody likes going to funerals do they? But I always think of him, I always remember him.

I think it was the doctors – the doctors wanted me to keep being active. I used to go to the gym to do a little exercise with Sarah and Catherine, the physios. They made a programme for me and I started all different activities. They asked me what I wanted to do, told me what was available and what I could fit in, like a school programme. That was five years ago when I was here – I only come here for sports now. So I've got a big connection with the centre really. When I'm not actually working, doing jobs here, I still communicate with the people here. Keep close with the people, the same people. I'm sort of supported. I feel supported with other people here, especially with the football team. It's people that I never knew before, but I got friendly with, made good friends, and we all just participated in sport. Family as well, they supported me since I was ill really. They used to come round, make sure I was up, when I went out with them they asked how I was. You know, just good friends really – just care.

I used to be so quiet, see, and shy. Now that I've got better I'm just talking and more relaxed – I feel better. And I focus better as well. Like when I used to answer the phone I used to stutter, get embarrassed. I was stuck for words. But now I'm just a different person. My mum's seen it as well, the change in me. I feel more confident when I'm speaking to somebody.

Since I was in Brentree I really feel on top of the world. Until I get an injury or something I don't want to stop really. I'm an active person, sports and interests – that's about it I suppose. It'll have to come to a halt when I get older, football-wise, I'll have to keep playing cricket and walking and just slow it down, don't do so much. But there's always cricket or something you can play when you get older.

The future? Well, I think it's looking quite bright. I'm optimistic. 'Cause you don't know what's gonna happen the day after do you? I could have a heart attack or something, anybody can, can't predict the day after can you? It's why you gotta make the most of the day you're doing now. You know, it's never tomorrow – you just gotta start today.

Our responses to the stories

We want to resist the temptation to analyse or summarise Laura and Colin's stories because, ultimately, stories are irreducible: no summary can do the work of the story. In other words, Laura and Colin's experiences are best expressed through the stories they chose to share. The stories in themselves offer many lessons about the benefits and provision of physical activity and mental health which may be damaged by further analysis on our part. Accordingly, we want to (as much as it is possible) allow the stories to 'speak for themselves' and encourage you, the reader, to draw your own conclusions in light of your own life experiences and professional circumstances. At the same time, we do not want to leave the stories 'hanging' without a response. This is because, as Frank (2005) notes, stories *call for* a response: a good story *invites* dialogue. It is in this spirit that we conclude the chapter by sharing *our* responses to Laura and Colin's stories in the form of a conversation between the two of us. By doing so, we each focus on certain issues within the stories that particularly resonated with our experiences – personal and professional. We invite you to reflect in a similar way – perhaps through engaging in dialogue with others who have read the stories – on the insights and meaning of Laura and Colin's stories in the context of your life.

Kitrina: I get a real sense of enthusiasm for sport in general and the joy of football, in particular, from Colin's story. He is a wonderful advocate for football!

David: Yes. The beginning section of his story reminds me of my grandfather, who was a professional footballer and cricketer. In the same way Colin does here, my grandfather used to tell stories of his long sport career – he seemed to be able to remember every detail of every game: the names, places, teams, results. I feel like I established some kind of connection with Colin from this part of his story, that there is common ground between him and my family. It left me with a strong sense of Colin as *being* a sportsman – his life seems to have always involved a connection with sport in terms of what he *does* and what he *talks about*. It seems to have been a constant across the years, from childhood to the present day.

Kitrina: Yes, in both Colin and Laura's stories, their current interests appear to align with the types of selves they created earlier in the story. Laura enjoyed dance and swimming as a child, and engages in these activities in adult life. Colin too had positive football experience as a child, and continues with this activity. The activities they described are somewhat gendered and stereotypical of what we expect males and females to be interested in – not *all* women like dance and swimming, and not *all* men like football. I wonder how we can better cater for those who fall outside the mainstream. I wonder how we as practitioners might challenge the stereotypes in order to make it possible for men to choose dance or women to join in with the football. I recognise that these aren't easy questions! I also share with both Colin and Laura their sense of whatever other problems there are in life, physical activity has something powerful to offer, not that it solves the problem or even reduces it, but it provides a sense of joy and fun in the moment.

David: Me too. I think that is probably why Laura's description of being injured and therefore prevented from taking part in sport and activity made a big impact for me. This section of the story got me thinking about my own physical activity, how much I rely on swimming, going to the gym, running or surfing on a day-to-day basis to feel well. I've thought before now how enforced inactivity would be a major problem for me because physical activity is something I feel I *need* on a daily basis. I am not sure how I'd get through life or deal with life's ups and downs without the freedom, joy, release that these forms of activity bring me. I've been very aware of a kind of double loss in several other participants' stories too – that on top of everything else mental health difficulties remove people from involvement in the sport or activity that is so important in their day-to-day life.

Kitrina: I was struck how both Laura and Colin remembered, in a positive way, *teachers* who made it possible for them each to enjoy an activity. Both remembered their swimming teachers and Laura also talked about her aerobics teacher. These positive memories underscore for me the importance of a good coach or teacher, in giving an individual confidence and facilitating success experiences.

David: Yes, and in terms of teaching or provision I really felt a big difference in Laura's description of the shift at the day centre from being *invited* to join an art group to being *prescribed* an art activity. Qualities like respect, empowerment and agency seem to be nurtured or preserved in the first instance and ignored, violated or destroyed in the second. I think I too would react badly to this change: for me it is often the *way* something is presented or suggested that makes the difference in how I feel about it in terms of motivation, attitude, my general disposition towards it. When I feel coerced, directed or channelled, I often end up resisting or rebelling against the intended outcome. Yet when I am *invited* I am more likely to feel positive, enthusiastic and willing.

Kitrina: I am *exactly* the same! And, related to that, both the stories underscored for me the importance of getting started at an appropriate level and in a supportive environment. In both stories, initial 'low level' activities paved the way for further physical activity groups. I wonder if this 'low level' is below what might be available in a community sport or activity session at a sport centre or health club. As we strive towards becoming more inclusive, I am concerned that the programmes on offer at most sports centres are still too intimidating for people who are experiencing the kind of difficulties Laura and Colin describe.

David: I think Laura's description of needing activity sessions which were 'less threatening' than what was available at the local sport centre sheds some light on that point. By using the metaphor of a computer running too many applications at one time, Laura communicates her need for simplified and well-managed sessions which offer a safe and predictable environment. It's interesting that Laura describes closely supported and manageable activity groups – where expectations are not set too high or too specific – as facilitating her later involvement in community-based groups and activities. Laura also articulates clearly the difficult issue of transition from activities in mental health settings to community, public or independent activity – describing how she experiences too many changes at once as threatening and likely to result in drop-out. When she talks about moving on from an activity group, Laura describes simultaneously losing a *familiar* activity environment, *friends* she has made through a particular activity group and the activity *itself*. This section of her story highlights a key issue in physical activity and sport provision: long-term sustainability.

Kitrina: But sometimes long-term sustainability may not be necessary! When Colin said: 'It was only a couple of weeks. After that I knew I'd had enough of it – that was enough of the gym for me I think. It did enough to boost my morale,' it made me think of our research with older women, many of whom said they found gyms boring. His comment reaffirmed for me the importance of doing something even when we *don't* intend to carry it on. In Colin's case, the gym provided an impetus to do something else that he *did* carry on. I see the same thing in Laura's story, when she talks about the badminton group providing the impetus to attend an aerobic session in a local authority sport centre. It made me remember how my parents gave me the same type of support to help me engage in badminton as a child, taking me to sessions, going in with me for the first few weeks, and encouraging me. Just because I no longer play badminton it doesn't mean those efforts were a waste of time! I can see from both stories how important these initial groups were for building confidence and knowledge in order to move on to other activities or groups.

David: That section of Colin's story contrasts so strongly with his account of being totally *inactive* during the acute phases of illness where he describes sleeping 'for hours and hours' and being 'so bored' in hospital. Even though I don't know what it is like to be a patient in a psychiatric hospital, this simple description helped me imagine *myself* there – what I might be like in this situation. The feeling of *just wanting to go to sleep* for me conjured up feelings of despair and defeat, of simply not being able to summon up the motivation to carry on. Although Colin didn't talk about those kinds of feelings explicitly, something in his descriptions evoked those thoughts in me. I suppose my response highlights how the work a story achieves is partly a result of what the reader brings to the story himself.

Kitrina: I was aware how Laura could story her life before and after her 'D-day' but remains unable to story the 'nasty blur' of acute mental health difficulties. We don't necessarily need to understand this time of her life to talk about her physical activity experiences, but I do wonder if we are perpetuating an absence of difficult (to hear and tell) stories by glossing over this part of her life. On the other hand, I also worry that talking about this period of her life might have adverse consequences for Laura.

David: I have felt the same and questioned whether or not it is right to explore painful and traumatic areas of a person's life in a research project. It's a difficult area to negotiate. It even relates to feeding back to participants following the interview. Some participants – and some mental health professionals too – have expressed a wish *not* to return to the stories or 'findings' which arose from the interviews.

Kitrina: When I asked Laura to read our version of her story she appeared quite hesitant and asked her partner to read it first. After her partner's response – 'Yes, that's you!' – Laura read the story and (after a few changes) was happy for it to be published. This in itself is a lesson to us that feeding back to participants can in certain circumstances be a dangerous path. Though we have an ethical imperative to share what we write about an individual, Laura showed me the importance of proceeding with caution and to consider whether there might be occasions when we should *not* feed back.

David: This is just one of so many complex issues which the stories raise – which can easily be glossed over through other research methods. Laura's story also brings complexity to the task of understanding mental illness and recovery. Things which are experienced as damaging by some others are described as helpful by Laura, and vice versa. For example, Patricia Deegan (1996, see chapter 1) describes being 'labelled' and diagnosed as an experience which harmed her sense of self, her identity, her hopes for the future. Laura, in contrast, describes this experience as helpful in that it 'made sense' of her psychological difficulties and facilitated access to treatment and financial support. This highlights the individual way in which mental health problems and treatment for those problems can be experienced, how recovery really is a very personal process. Complexity is present too in Laura's description of appearing from the outside to be a 'high-flier', to be 'well' and flourishing, yet secretly so *unwell*. This section made a real impact on me. I see – and feel – cultural pressures to 'achieve' in terms of career or money that sometimes seem to compromise my own sense of peace and balance. Sometimes for me, too, the apparently 'doing well' periods aren't particularly happy or healthy ones – I've often felt more 'well' during what might from the outside be seen as 'down time'. This might be why I find the later part of Laura's story to be so powerful, the part when she describes moving from being stuck within 'society's straitjacket' to being able to 'blossom in a different way'. I love the sense of transformation she describes: a sense of breaking free or getting outside social expectations and pressures, to live authentically according to a different set of values. The final paragraph of Colin's story is similarly powerful to me. Several times when I've been reading the story to an audience at a conference or during a lecture, I've found myself choking up on these closing lines. There is something deep and profound here – yet I don't quite know what. I wonder if it is beauty: a sense of optimism and hope that is present after or through the difficulty and challenge of mental illness. I wonder if it is simply the sound of truth.

Kitrina: It certainly contrasts very strongly with the part of her story where Laura describes being known within the hospital as 'number 14'.

David: Yes. And when Laura talked about how she felt psych services saw her as a 'problem' rather than a 'person', that made me think back to young people I have worked with as a teacher, those students whose lives have been marked by difficulty, hardship or abuse from a young age. It was so easy for me to see these individuals – within a class of 30-odd 10- and 11-year-olds – as a 'problem', largely because the educational system *we* have set up fails to provide them with an environment in which they can function or fit. How easy it is for me – and *all* the teachers, the school system – to write them off as failures without their possibilities ever being seen. Without giving people who are experiencing problems or difficulties a chance, what hope do they have to be something more?

Kitrina: It makes me wonder in what ways I may act similarly with people who I conduct research with or teach. Laura's story made me consider how I might evaluate or see people at a particular point in their life without regard to their past, without the benefit of knowing the person. It forces me to remember that I need to guard against letting my expectations or behaviour towards a person be controlled by first impressions.

David: At this point in my life, I also find myself reflecting on the section of Colin's story where he describes how he 'keeps close with the people' he has known through sport. Care and support through these relationships seem to have been so important to him. These are relationships he has established through his long-term involvement in sport and physical activity. Modern life and making a career – these things sometimes seem to have conspired in my life to threaten the kinds of relationships which Colin describes. It makes me wonder how I would cope in a time of hardship having distanced myself from family and social networks by moving 200 miles across the country for a job. It leads me to wonder what we might do to help those people who *don't* have this kind of supportive social structure around them when they experience mental health problems.

Rebuilding identity through sport and physical activity

4

With time and experience, everyone develops a sense of who they are: this sense of self is profoundly challenged and fragmented by the experience of mental health problems. Within each person who has faced mental health problems there remains a persistent, healthy self trying to survive. But this is all too easily eclipsed by the identity of 'mental patient', which tends to mask all other identities.

Julie Repper and Rachel Perkins (2003, p. 49)[1]

At the first session of a golf programme we initiated for a group of people with severe mental health difficulties (see Carless & Douglas, 2004, 2009c; chapter 11), we were surprised that several individuals arrived wearing golf clothing, carrying a golf ball or other piece of golf equipment. As we made our introductions we saw that although some individuals had no background in golf, others seemed keen to show their knowledge of golf by using golf terminology or name-checking top golfers. Reflecting later on this first session, we realised that these objects, clothing and talk were biographical markers (Dant, 2001) which tell us something about the identities of these individuals.

As we began to explore the meaning of golf in the participants' lives, we learned that, for some at least, the experience of mental illness had resulted in the fracture of a valued component of their identity: an *athletic identity*. In this chapter we explore the ways in which re-involvement in sport and physical activity can contribute to recovery through facilitating the recovery of this component of identity. To do so we focus in detail on the life story of one participant named Ben (see Carless, 2008), whose identity and sense of self has, for most of his life, been intricately tied to sport and exercise

---

[1] This excerpt was published in *Social Inclusion and Recovery*, by Julie Repper and Rachel Perkins. Copyright Elsevier 2003. Reprinted with permission.

in general and running in particular. Ben's stories and experiences, we hope, illustrate one way through which sport and physical activity can contribute to recovery in the context of mental illness.

'I got the running bug': forming an athletic identity

Brewer and colleagues (1993, pp. 237–8) define athletic identity as 'the degree to which an individual identifies with the athletic role' and suggest that 'the individual with a strong athletic identity ascribes great importance to involvement in sport/exercise'. They describe athletic identity as a social role which is influenced by family members, friends, coaches, teachers and the media. While an identity defines who we are or who we want to be, it also grounds us within a social group and provides a sense of belonging. One doesn't need to look further than the amount of sports coverage on television and in newspapers to see that sport is highly valued and socially significant in Western society. Besides revealing an interest and enthusiasm for sport, the presence of an athletic identity also therefore signals a person's sense of connection with a socially significant and valued set of activities and roles.

Ben's stories of his life portray the development of an athletic identity at a young age when sport became a valued and meaningful component of his life and suggest that his athletic identity was shaped by socio-cultural factors. The following excerpt, in which Ben describes the role his brother played in him coming to regard himself as a 'skilful' footballer, provides an illustration:

> In school I was always a fast runner. I was a real, I'm really skilful at football, real good footballer. My brother could have been a professional, he was really skilful, and he taught me when I was in my first year in seniors. He taught me all the moves and this enabled me to be from a below average player to a really good player 'cause of the moves he taught me. I was fast anyway, to be a really good player you gotta be fast and skilful, it's gotta be two ... So that's what I did – he taught me the moves and I became a real, good, skilful footballer.

Describing his memories of this period of his life, Ben spoke passionately of the importance of football. He described how 'I was always playing football from the age of 16 ... we lived for football' and recounted his experiences of playing local league football in the adult league even though he was still only 16. It was a few years later that Ben started running as a way of training for football. As he put it: 'I think what really got me into exercise was probably the fact that I was a footballer. I sort of used the jogging to help with the football.' Over the following years Ben increasingly became involved in running, a process that was also culturally influenced as he was exposed to marathons on television:

> I'd seen the marathons on telly. I thought, 'I'll have a go at them!' I did it with my mate like, we went out running round Dilsley Common. That's when I got the running bug then, got through the pain barrier and we were running every day then, running miles. But I always kept in with football. In 1988 I did a 6-miler, and from 1990 I done a few half marathons, and from 1992 to 93 I did a few 20-milers.

As these examples indicate, Ben's recollections of his childhood and young adult life – long before his mental health difficulties began – portray sport and exercise (particularly football and running) as important aspects of his identity and sense of self. In view of what was to come, it is notable that Ben's stories of this period in his life demonstrate a degree of narrative coherence, agency and continuity in that they portray physical activity as:

(1) bringing a sense of meaning and purpose to his life;
(2) allowing some degree of personal control; and
(3) a constant in his life.

'Out of control': a descent into chaos

Ben was in his late twenties when he was first prescribed antipsychotic medication to treat symptoms of paranoia. Over a seven-year period his medical records detail a total of fourteen hospital admissions, three of which were extended inpatient periods at a psychiatric hospital. During this time Ben's mental health is noted to have fluctuated considerably – his medical records document periods of 'extreme anxiety and desperation' and 'extremely negative and suicidal thoughts' interspersed with periods of improvement and remission. Over the years Ben was treated with electro-convulsive therapy and it is recorded that four antipsychotic and two antidepressant medications were tried and rejected on the basis of side effects which, according to an entry in his medical records, he found to be 'unacceptable'. While the medication was reported to reduce his psychotic symptoms, serious side effects (such as tremor, pacing and blunted affect in addition to significant weight gain) were noted. By the time Ben reached his mid-thirties, his medical records state that the psychotic symptoms had stabilised and that an 'acceptable' medication regime had been found which resulted in fewer side effects. Although he was subsequently discharged from hospital to a residential unit, Ben was recorded to still be experiencing what were described as 'continual' anxiety attacks which could last up to eight hours.

During one interview Ben recounted memories of how his mental health difficulties began:

> When I first started getting unwell I had a paranoia illness, psychosis. Thinking people were following me and stuff like that. 'Cause it was brought on, it was brought on by too much stress and failure. I had a lot of things go wrong with me, lot of, you know, sort of marriage breakup and, uh, I failed, I had a lot of failures and stuff so that made me, and I had all that on board, and it sort of spiralled out of control … It all built up. I just got worse and worse and in the end, *[clicks fingers]* bang! I just had a nervous breakdown.

In this description Ben depicts the time around the onset of mental illness as a time during which he gradually lost control of his life and descended into an increasingly chaotic existence. Feelings of a loss of control, sense of confusion and lack of under-standing are also present in Ben's description of an anxiety (panic) attack:

> Well it's a fear of a fear really. You're just frightened and you don't know why. Everything, everything becomes out of touch. You're just frightened to death for some reason and you don't know why. That's what it's like. And it lasts for, lasts about an hour something like that. Then it's gone again. And then you think, well you know, what was I worried about?

According to Clive Baldwin (2005), severe mental illness is a threat to narrative agency in that it can remove the ability and opportunity to author one's own life story. The lack of agency in Ben's stories of this time is particularly marked when compared to the sense of personal control that was evident in his descriptions of his earlier involvement in football and running. When talking about exercise, Ben tells a story of relative personal control; when talking about mental illness, he tells an 'out of control' story. In this sense, Ben's stories of becoming unwell suggest he lost narrative agency (i.e. he became unable to author his own life story) as the chaotic, out-of-control conditions of psychotic illness took over his life, displacing his earlier sport and exercise stories. This abrupt change in Ben's stories also represents a potentially prob-lematic breakdown in narrative continuity (Baldwin, 2005) in that exercise and sport, which had previously been constants in Ben's life story, were no longer the focus of his stories.

For a period of four years, when his mental health was at its lowest level, Ben was involved in no sport or exercise whatsoever. During this time he was, in his words, 'smoking about, at least, 20 cigarettes a day' and, according to his medical records, drinking heavily at times. He was also receiving antipsychotic medication, a side effect of which can be significant weight gain (Green *et al.*, 2000). Ben described how 'I was on the wrong medication – the medication was making me worse. It made me put on a lot of weight and I couldn't do exercise anyway I was so overweight. I went up to 21 stone.' In terms of physical fitness, he was at an all-time low: 'I was so out of condition. I was walking up Winbridge field with Rob, I had to keep lying down I was so unfit.'

For Andrew Sparkes (1997, p. 101), 'the problem of identity is the problem of arriving at a life story that makes sense (provides unity and purpose) within a sociohistorical matrix that embodies a much larger story'. In this light, we see that when Ben's previous exercise-focused life story was replaced by the 'much larger story' of mental illness, it became impossible to sustain an athletic identity as talking about exercise or sport participation simply did not 'fit' his lived experience at this time. As Gergen and Gergen (2006) observe, it is difficult or impossible to sustain a story which is entirely at odds with one's lived experience. We suggest that a central aspect of Ben's identity and sense of self was thereby lost – along with a way to find purpose and meaning in his life through involvement in sport and exercise.

The tone and form of Ben's stories at this time are akin to a *chaos narrative* where 'stories are chaotic in their absence of narrative order. Events are told as the storyteller experiences life: without consequences or discernible causality' (Frank, 1995, p. 97). Chaos stories are not unusual in the context of serious illness and it may be that, as Brendan Stone (2006) suggests, severe mental disturbance is not in itself amenable to portrayal in the form of a coherent narrative. In other words, as Frank (1995) suggests, when living in chaos reflection and coherent storytelling are impossible. While Ben was able to describe the onset of mental illness and his experience of an anxiety attack during our interviews, a sense of understanding and coherence is likely to have been possible only because the events he was describing happened some time before. In other words, it is only because he has had time to reflect on these events that Ben is able to create a coherent story of this period of time.

'Back running again': towards restitution

It was seven years after the onset of mental illness that Ben first re-engaged in exercise while attending a vocational rehabilitation day centre. His initial exercise took the form of one-to-one sessions with a physiotherapist in a makeshift gym at a day centre. Preliminary assessments of his exercise programme were promising: a 'much improved mental state' is noted in his records alongside improved fitness, weight loss, and that he had quit smoking and was happy about these changes. Two years after starting at the day centre Ben was documented to have experienced psychological, social and physical improvements and reported feeling generally well although panic attacks continued to occur about once a week. Ben believed that finding the 'right' medication, in a dose that combined clinical effectiveness with acceptable side effects, was a necessary prerequisite for him to re-engage in exercise. He described how at this time:

> I was on the right medication, I felt better and I thought to myself, well, I'll get back into running again and keeping fit again ... I got well enough to start exercising again. Because I wasn't well enough to carry on with the exercise, I became so unwell that I couldn't do it. And then I had no interest in it.

This desire to 'get back' into running was repeatedly raised during our interviews. For example, Ben described his return to running:

> I started getting fitter and fitter and eventually I was back to, apart from being overweight, I was back to normal again ... back to what I used to be like ... The first time I was out running again I felt on top of the world – I was actually back to what I used to be like doing running again.

When Ben states that by running 'I was back to normal again ... back to what I used to be like' he tells a *restitution narrative*; a story which centres on a return to wellness, of striving for a 'cure'. Arthur Frank (1995) characterises restitution stories as focusing on returning the ill person to health and relying on metaphors like 'as good as new'. Ben tells a restitution story when he says 'It's just having the right medication and the right frame of mind and exercising – you can totally get cured of a mental illness I reckon.' By telling a *successful* restitution story, Ben is able to replace the earlier chaos stories (of his experience of psychotic illness) with a more optimistic or hopeful story about getting back to health. Hence, by returning to running Ben is engaging in an activity which he believes has the potential to provide a 'cure' but also – perhaps more importantly – successfully reconnecting with a central and valued element of his previous self. This element is his athletic identity.

Sparkes (1997, pp. 101–2) writes that 'As individuals construct past events and actions in personal narratives they engage in a dynamic process of claiming identities and constructing lives.' Through starting to run once more, not only was Ben *doing* the activity itself, but he was also able to legitimately create and share *stories* about his running in day-to-day interactions. In line with Sparkes's point above, this process – through which running stories resumed an authentic place within his life story – allowed Ben to reinstate narrative continuity and reclaim his previous athletic identity which was fractured during the psychotic stages of mental illness. Baldwin (2005) suggests that efforts to maintain narrative continuity are a necessary component of service provision in order to help people preserve valued aspects of their past lives through the present and into the future. It is primarily through re-involvement in exercise that Ben was able to achieve this task.

'Things become brighter': beyond restitution

Although Ben tells a restitution story when he describes exercise as a 'cure' for mental illness or as a way to 'get back' to life before mental illness, there is also another side to his experience of physical activity, as the following excerpt illustrates:

> When I'm exercising it makes you feel up for it, it makes you feel good about yourself as well. When I'm actually exercising no matter what I feel like I don't feel depressed or anything – I always feel good, no matter, when I'm exercising, just makes me feel good.

Within this description is a portrayal of *positive* experiences gained through running. This perspective was also communicated when Ben described further how running affected him psychologically:

> You think more when you're running, I think. You can work things out. Things that are bad don't seem that bad anyway ... Things become brighter, you know what I mean ... things sort of, you see things more clear and everything around looks brighter ... I suppose it makes you face the problem head on. It makes you feel as though it's not that bad in the first place – there's nothing really to worry about.

William Anthony (1993) suggests that mental health interventions can do more than remove impairment and dysfunction; that they can also bring success and purpose to a person's life. Inherent within Ben's stories is a sense of running making a positive contribution to his life in this way. Thus, through running it was not so much that Ben was left with *fewer* symptoms and dysfunction, but that he experienced *more* good feelings, optimism, confidence, success and satisfaction with his life. It seems to us that involvement in exercise brought something *positive* to Ben's life, and these things were valuable and meaningful to him irrespective of the extent to which exercise alleviated the symptoms of mental illness.

By talking about the presence of positive experiences, Ben's descriptions move from a restitution narrative towards a *quest narrative*. According to Frank (1995), tellers of quest stories construe illness as the occasion for a journey that becomes a quest. In his words, 'What is quested for may never be wholly clear, but the quest is defined by the ill person's belief that something is to be gained through the experience' (p. 115).

One of the most striking aspects of our interviews was the way Ben considered that his experiences had changed him in some way. Despite the hardships and difficulties he experienced through ten years of serious mental illness, treatments and numerous hospitalisations, Ben described how he had come to value life more as a result of his experiences. While talking about his previous lifestyle when he was unwell, which included smoking and heavy drinking, Ben said, 'I think the exercise and the illness has made me value life more and I won't touch another drink again, I'll never ever get drunk again ... or smoke. Fitness for me now is a way of life.' Here Ben once again signals the importance of exercise in his identity and sense of self: because he valued exercise as a 'way of life' he was able to rationalise his decision to quit drinking and smoking on the basis that both would adversely affect his running.

Frank (1995) describes how the quest narrative tells self-consciously of being transformed through an illness experience, a process which is evident in both the preceding excerpt and Ben's description of a further change that occurred as a result of his experiences:

> Having a mental illness wakens you up. You realise then that things you worried about in the past, you think hang on a minute, I'm not worrying about that again 'cause it makes me ill. So I either stop worrying about it or ... I make myself ill again. So you don't worry about it.

By describing positive change – but not denying the severe symptoms and experiences he has been through – Ben's stories have something in common with quest stories told by some cancer survivors (see Frank, 1995) and connect with Peter Chadwick's (2009, p. 6) assertion that 'Psychotic illness can at times be a creative illness ... there are occasions when patients not only get well, they go on to become better still with time such that they become better than they were before.' Likewise, Ben's experiences connect with Anthony's (1993) conception of recovery as sometimes occurring independent of symptom relief. In Anthony's (1993, p. 21) terms, although a person may still experience major episodes of symptom exacerbation, she or he might have 'significantly restored task or role performance and/or removed significant opportunity barriers. From a recovery perspective, those successful outcomes may have led to the growth of new meaning and purpose in one's life.' Ben's stories suggest that he successfully recreated a sense of meaning and purpose in his life and – to a considerable extent – he did so through involvement in running.

'I can't beat it': the limits of restitution

Anxiety (panic) attacks were a debilitating and ongoing aspect of Ben's illness. During the earlier stages, these attacks occurred seemingly at random, forcing him to abandon whatever activity he was doing at the time. By the time our research took place, the attacks had changed in nature in that they only occurred when Ben was running. According to a clinical psychologist's entry in Ben's medical records, 'The attacks seem to occur only on the treadmill in the gym and at a certain point when he is out running. There seems to be a mixture of physiological arousal and "paranoid" ideas.' Ben described the occurrence of an anxiety attack during a recent race:

> I had it in that half marathon. Not only was I thinking of keeping going, I had to deal with a panic attack as well – on the run. So I went 13 miles and I was in the panic attack all the way round. I got out of it as I, as I finished and had a shower, and as I was in the shower it just disappeared. I was alright.

At this point in time, the most debilitating symptom of Ben's mental illness – an anxiety attack – was now occurring *only* when he engaged in the activity he loved. On the one hand, involvement in running allowed him to maintain an athletic identity and provided valued psychological benefits, while on the other it seemed to threaten his mental health. This turn of events led a clinical psychologist to question whether Ben's running had become an addiction that was doing more harm than good. A key consideration in this regard is the ways in which Ben's anxiety attacks had changed over the years. Although in the past the attacks had been seemingly random, uncontrollable, debilitating and had lasted up to eight hours in duration, his medical records documented how, more recently, his 'panic attacks continue generally when running ... but he is able to continue running through the attack'. As such, the attacks had become more predictable (in that they most often occurred when he ran), shorter in duration (less than one hour), and Ben was reportedly learning to control them so that they did not interrupt his activities. Literally, Ben was now able to *run through* an anxiety attack.

Ben described his strategy for coping with an attack while running:

> Well sometimes if I can divert my thought I'll be OK. All I gotta do is divert my thought. But it's hard to do. You gotta try and take your mind off it for a few seconds and then [clicks fingers] it's gone. But it's just chatting to other runners – sometimes it'll go, like, chatting to them, other times it'll stay ... I gotta try and concentrate on focusing on not having the attack – just getting round all the race ... I can get through it sometimes. Other times I need to lay down, I can't beat it.

In this excerpt, Ben describes the occurrence of a psychotic episode which, in his words, 'I can't beat.' At this time, by his own admission, there is no cure and restitution is not possible. When this happens, Frank (1995) suggests, an alternative story is needed to avoid *narrative wreckage* and the re-emergence of chaos.

It is, we think, the availability of a quest narrative – in the form of stories about the meaning, value and transformative potential of exercise – which allows Ben to avoid narrative wreckage. The following excerpt provides an illustration of this kind of story:

> I suppose in a way it (exercise) is a bit of a drug like – want to do it to get that good feeling back again ... I think it's better actually than drinking. I think drinking, you're living in a dream world. That's what I reckon. You're dependent on it ... 'cause at the end of the day after you stop drinking you've gotta come back to reality, can't drink all your life. But if you're keeping fit, it's free, you don't have to pay for it you can just do it 'cause you like doing it. You're not living in a dream world, you're actually feeling better – making yourself feel better ... Other people might get a kick out of other things, but for me it's exercise.

Within this account, exercise is portrayed as a kind of quest: a quest to *feel good*, a quest for fitness, and a quest over which Ben has some degree of control. Through storying exercise in this way, Ben is able to preserve narrative coherence, continuity and agency even when the restitution story fails. He does so, we suggest, by drawing on a quest narrative which, according to Frank (1995), speaks from the ill person's perspective and holds chaos at bay.

Key points

- Ben's life history provides several insights into how sport or physical activity involvement can be psychologically beneficial for a person with a strong athletic identity. It reveals how: (i) serious mental illness can disrupt a pre-existing athletic identity, removing agency, continuity and coherence from a person's life story; (ii) through re-engaging in exercise it is possible for a person to rebuild or reclaim their athletic identity; (iii) exercise and sport can provide an arena in which an individual with an athletic identity may regain control of their life story and rebuild their identity in the wake of serious mental illness. Ben's story therefore suggests that exercise can contribute to recovery by being a personally meaningful activity which reinforces identity and sense of self.
- Not everyone will benefit from sport or physical activity in this way – these kinds of benefits are most likely to be experienced by people who show signs of holding a strong athletic identity. Potential 'signals' of an athletic identity include: a strong interest in sport/exercise; regular conversations about sport/exercise; wearing sports clothing (such as football shirts etc.); owning sports equipment or memorabilia. In our experience, we have found that men in particular often display signs of an athletic identity which may be beneficially developed or reinforced through sport or exercise involvement.
- An athletic identity, for some individuals, might be understood in the terms of narrative therapy as a *preferred identity*. Narrative theory – as well as Ben's story – suggests that if an individual is able to nurture and develop their preferred identity many psychological benefits become possible, not least the ability to resist dominant and potentially damaging externally imposed meta-narratives (and identities) such as the chaos narrative or the medical narrative.
- Research in sport (e.g. Sparkes, 1998; Douglas & Carless, 2006, 2009a; Carless & Douglas, 2009a) has shown that psychological dangers exist when an athletic identity becomes dominant to the extent that it eclipses all other identities and roles. On the basis of this research, it is important that alternative stories and identities are also allowed space and are supported (as we discuss in chapters 7 and 8).

Implications

- For some individuals, involvement in sport and physical activity is crucial to psychological well-being because it is a valued dimension of their identity and sense of self. Practitioners, health professionals and coaches need to understand that for people like this, it is not the case that *any* form of activity or sport will be beneficial. Rather, it is more likely that a *specific* activity or sport will be meaningful to a particular individual – in the preceding example the sport that was meaningful to Ben was running. It is therefore important that practitioners take time to discover the particular sport or exercise form/s that are meaningful and valued by the individual and tailor provision on this basis. Sensitivity and awareness of the individual's preferences seems critical.

- It is unusual for a person who has experienced severe mental health difficulties to achieve an immediate return to their former identity or their previous level of sport/exercise performance. As Ben's story reveals, this process is likely to take place over an extended period of time. It is therefore important to avoid considering sport or exercise initiatives a failure if an individual drifts in and out of involvement or drops out of one activity to pursue another. Small steps, patience and open-mindedness are needed.

- For a person with an athletic identity, progression and improvement may be particularly important because sport or exercise milestones are likely to hold particular meaning and significance. On this basis, practitioners might consider liaising with each individual in terms of her or his sport/exercise aspirations. What does the person want to achieve through activity? What are the person's hopes for future involvement? The opportunity to be involved in or work towards awards or certificates of ability; tournaments, leagues or competitions; coaching qualifications; the organisation of sport events are examples of potentially meaningful achievements for a person with an athletic identity.

Action, achievement and relationships

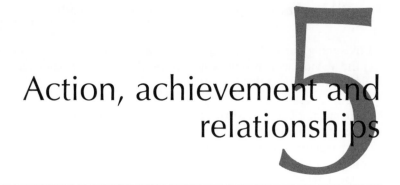

Did you ever wonder how it is we imagine the world in the way we do, how it is we imagine ourselves, if not through our stories?

Thomas King (2008, p. 15)

In the previous chapter we focused on the way in which involvement in sport or physical activity can facilitate recovery for a person with an athletic identity through rebuilding or recreating identity and sense of self. But how might sport and exercise help in the recovery of people who do not hold an athletic identity, those individuals who may not have a positive sport or physical activity history? In this chapter we turn our attention to this question by analysing data – in the form of stories and accounts recorded in interview transcripts and field notes – collected during our research with a group of people experiencing severe and enduring mental health problems (see Carless & Douglas, 2008a).

By exploring these stories in detail, we seek to answer two specific questions:

(1) What are the key characteristics of the talk and interactions which related to sport and physical activity participation?
(2) How might these characteristics contribute to recovery in the context of mental illness?

In response to the first question, we describe three narrative types which were repeatedly evident within individuals' accounts of their sport and exercise experiences. We term these *action*, *achievement* and *relationship* narratives and suggest that these story types provide insight into how sport and physical activity can be experienced as psychologically beneficial by people who use mental health services. In response to the second question, we offer an interpretation of the three story types in relation to current theory and research regarding the ways that recovery necessitates the recreation of a sense of meaning, purpose and identity.

An action narrative: 'going places and doing stuff'

> I like going out and about, like I said, people, you know, having a soft drink and stuff, playing with people, enjoy yourself ... keeping your mind busy, it's going places and doing stuff.

A recurring motif around which participants' talk about their sport and physical activity involvement was structured is the concept of *action*. By 'action' we mean, in the words of the participant above, 'going places and doing stuff'. In this regard, the action narrative centred on *embodied experience* – some kind of physical process or bodily movement which was enacted by the individual. For some, taking action – having something to do and somewhere to go – was expressed as being personally valuable and meaningful even if only to the extent that it gave them a reason to get out of the house:

> It's just that I've got an activity for the afternoon that I'm not sat watching TV something like that. I watch so much it just sort of draws me. I need to sort of break away from a day indoors and get out and do something ... It's something to get me out of bed, get out of bed that morning.

We think that the action narrative is significant in that it differs markedly from dominant stories – the meta-narrative – of mental illness which tend to revolves around *inactivity*; of not doing much and not having much to do, of withdrawing from life (see Deegan, 1996; Smith, 1999; Baker-Brown, 2006; Stone, 2009). One participant, for example, described his experience of hospitalisation in a psychiatric ward: 'I was just bored in there – nothing to do. I didn't do much. I was so bored. I didn't hardly do nothing. I just stayed in the ward and just went to bed and that was it.' Similarly, stories of other phases of illness were commonly characterised by inactivity: 'Over at my mother's house I used to go to sleep a lot. I just switched off like ... I used to sleep for hours and hours.'

Participants told how taking action affected them in positive ways. One young man, for example, told how playing football (and even being *involved* with football) provided a more positive focus for his thoughts because at these times:

> my mind's occupied. I think other things. I don't really think about bad things that I might think about if I wasn't doing something ... It can happen with other things but I think sport is such an active thing it tends to have that effect on me.

Other participants' action stories portray them as 'keeping busy' through involvement in sport and exercise. The importance of this is illustrated in the following exchange:

> Depression was my main problem. I suffered from depression and a bit of stress like. I think when I was young I overdone it ... and what with our dad passing away as well like, that was another bout of depression I had as well like, went to the funeral and that sort of turned it on again like, you know ... but I feel good now. I feel OK now.

Kitrina: What do you think has been able to change that?
Uh [pause]. Doing activities I think is the main thing – keeps me busy, you know.

Another individual elaborated on how keeping busy through sport and exercise gave him the feeling that he was making good use of his time. Referring to his involvement with a five-a-side football group, he said:

> I enjoy it, have a sense of satisfaction that I actually played because I was doing something with my time. That's important I think – to actually be able to use your time properly … I know I haven't wasted my time, I've used my time constructively, doing something that'll do me good.

For him, 'using time properly' related to his belief that, through participating in sport and physical activity, he was engaging in an activity that would provide valued physical and psychological health benefits.

For those individuals who maintained their involvement, sport and exercise activities came to be a valued part of their weekly or daily routine or schedule. Referring to a community-based five-a-side league in which he had become involved, one participant remarked that,

> It's a routine you get used to I think. It's like football, I get excited about football on a Monday. When you turn up there and watch other people play before you go on there, you get confident and you look forward to participating in the game.

For some who voluntarily took part in sport and exercise groups, there was a sense that, in addition to being 'used', time passed quickly. In this sense there was a perception among some participants that through taking action and doing things, time sped up, that they no longer felt that they had endless time on their hands. A short exchange between two members of a nine-week golf programme, documented in our field notes, communicates a feel for this view:

> Andrew went on to remark that 'These sessions seem to have gone ever so quickly.' Peter agreed, 'Yeah. I can't believe it's been two months since we started.' (David, 16 July)

In this regard, sport and physical activity was experienced by some as a 'good' way to use one's time, as an activity through which time passes quickly. One such individual went as far as to describe an afternoon playing golf at a local municipal course as 'the best birthday I could have asked for'.

An achievement narrative: 'that was way better than I ever thought I would have done'

A second type of narrative which was evident in participants' stories we term an *achievement* narrative. The *Concise Oxford English Dictionary* defines the verb *achieve* as to 'bring about or accomplish by effort, skill or courage'. Central to the achievement narrative were descriptions, accounts and stories that encapsulate this definition, describing or reliving instances of accomplishment and success which resulted from effort, skill or courage. One individual, for example, told an achievement story in the context of long-distance running:

> I went with a physio and done the Milwood 10k [a local race] not last year the year before, [we] both ran round together ... That was good, gave me something to aim for. I stopped last time. I stopped in the Buxham as well. But this year I never stopped at all, I got all the way round on the Buxham and the Milwood. So that's an achievement isn't it?

Importantly, achievement brought a range of positive feelings such as a sense of satisfaction from learning and performing skills:

> Well, I get satisfaction from playing football. If I score a goal I'm pleased with myself and it gives satisfaction that way. Even if I didn't score a goal, some weeks when I haven't scored, when I played well in defence or midfield ... football skills like trapping the ball, bringing it down and controlling the football and passing it using your alertness.

For others, a sense of achievement related to seeing their skills improve which subsequently increased their enjoyment of the activity as the following exchange illustrates:

David: How do you feel about your own play?
Well today it was brilliant because I got two threes and I can't ever remember getting that. [laughs]
David: Do you feel you've changed over the two months at all in terms of golf?
Hmmm [in a tone suggesting agreement] [pause]
David: What's changed?
Um [pause], I just think it's got more enjoyable as it's gone on.
David: What's that down to then?
Getting a couple of threes! [laughs]

Through participant observation we witnessed the way in which achievements resulted in displays of pleasure and satisfaction in individuals which were often shared with others in the activity group. A change in mood and demeanour, as a result of a good putting performance, is evident in the following description taken from our field notes:

> In the second group, of Jerry, Peter and Harry, it was Harry who particularly seemed pleased with his successes. Having been noticeably quiet in the café [beforehand], mostly looking down from under the peak of his cap towards the ground, he looked up, cheered and beamed a broad smile following his first 50 point score. (David, 4 June)

Achievements for some, we suggest, related to positive feelings which were directly connected to an embodied sense of proficient movement, feel or outcome. One participant, for example, described how making a good golf shot resulted in positive sensations of which he was clearly aware and which he found enjoyable:

Kitrina: How does it make you feel when you hit the good shots?

Oh, lovely … yeah, feels good. You know that you can do it, like. It gives you a bit of satisfaction … when you connect with the ball, when you follow through with the ball, and the club, you make contact with the ball, it's that sort of swing like, and when you know you hit it – it's that sound as well I think, you know, there's a good sound.

Another individual linked his increasing competence at golf to a sense of optimism and hope concerning his ongoing improvement:

Playing the round today, I enjoyed it as far as I got. I started to get some slightly better scores, that didn't seem fluke-ish … I feel that I'm making improvement and there's no reason why, if I carry on, I can't improve my game.

Thus, achievements in the present often generalised to optimism and confidence regarding future activity. As one participant put it, 'When you hit the ball, if you do something right, it gives you confidence, you feel as if you could do it again. You get that feeling you could do it again.'

Notwithstanding the challenges of learning new technical skills which any beginner will face, participants often came to perceive themselves as competent, skilled and proficient at sport-related skills. This is illustrated by one participant's description of his own golf ability:

I know how to drive the ball, definitely, down a fairway. Cause I've done that quite a few times at the pitch and putt … That's probably one thing I like about it – the driving shots I play. I get good distance on my driving shots … When I'm driving, I think about distance and length – it's a good tip that for the serious golfer.

In this remark, the individual identifies himself as a competent and 'serious' golfer. In so doing, he associates himself with both the culture of golf and with other golfers. This is potentially significant in that he is thereby able to tell a story about his life which revolves around achievement, success and 'being good at' a specific activity which is culturally accepted and endorsed by others. In telling this story, he is able to incorporate 'being a golfer' within his identity and sense of self and – for this individual at least – this self-identification is positive because he values golf and considers it to be a worthwhile activity. Thus, in creating and telling an achievement story in the context of a popular sport, he has a story which is shared *by* – and can potentially be shared *with* – many others in society.

A recurring motif within individual achievement stories was a sense of *surprise* at one's own achievements. This was particularly evident among members of the golf group who either had never played golf before or who had not played since the onset of mental illness. As one individual put it, 'I was surprised I could do it at all … when I hit the ball I was amazed that it went anywhere.' In this regard, participants' achievements frequently exceeded their own self-expectations as the following exchange illustrates:

Kitrina: Can you tell me about the most memorable shots that you've hit?
Yes. One, was it a week or a couple of weeks ago, where I putted and unexpectedly got the ball into the hole! … I couldn't believe it, what I saw … I felt chuffed – with disbelief!

Likewise, another participant described being 'amazed' by his most memorable golf shot:

> I hit a lovely one last week with the six iron, you know, when we were out at [names pitch and putt course] ... on the first one – I couldn't believe it! I thought 'How the hell did I do that?' like. I thought, well I've got to try and remember what I'd actually done to hit that ball ... just sort of prepared for the shot, I just swung the club and it worked and I thought 'Oh, hurray!' like. Yeah, thought, you know, I've done it like ... It was amazing, I amazed myself really. I thought it wasn't going to work out that way.

These moments of surprise were not unusual. Frequently, as the following excerpt from our field notes illustrates, the pleasure and surprise at one's own successful performance prompted verbal interaction between the group members thus constituting a shared moment of celebration:

> There was a great sense of excitement also among several individuals. Harry regularly called out excitedly, 'Whoa! It's on the green!' while Andrew several times gasped 'Ooooh!' in response to his better shots. On the first hole, following a fairway shot, Andrew exclaimed, 'Hey! That was *way* better than I *ever* thought I would have done!' (David, 9 July)

On reflection, it seemed to us that some of the participants had few – if any – positive expectations concerning their ability to achieve success in activities or tasks. A widespread sense of surprise when one's activities or tasks *did* go well or *were* successful has some troubling connotations regarding the possible life experiences and biographies of these individuals. As Repper and Perkins (2003) point out, it is not unusual for a combination of previous adverse life experiences *and* negative expectations held by others (e.g. mental health professionals, family members, friends, the public, other service users) to lead to a loss of confidence in one's own abilities and, eventually, a loss of hope regarding the outcomes of future activities. It is on this basis that the experience of *success* in physical activity or sport – and, importantly, being able to re-live and share those experiences through achievement stories – can play a valuable role in supporting recovery.

A relationship narrative: 'sharing a common thing'

> Well you're meeting other people that are sharing a common thing aren't you really? Common exercises, sharing that experience. That's what I reckon anyway. So it's good on that side of it ... all doing the same thing, got the same experience and got something to talk about.

The third type of narrative evident in participants' talk about sport and exercise we characterise as a *relationship* narrative. As the excerpt above suggests, shared experience and interaction with others were hallmarks of these stories. For several participants, it was the opportunity of a social time with others – being with and sharing time and/or an activity with other people – that served as their primary motive for sport and exercise. This is illustrated in the following exchange:

David: So, have you played any golf before?
No. I have never played golf in my life. This is the first time.
David: Do you watch it on TV?
No, I'd get bored.
David: So no interest in golf?
Not interested in golf, not really.
David: So why did you decide to join this group?
'Cause there's a lot of people – the social – you can enjoy. Otherwise, I'm bored, do
    you understand me? There's people there, that's what I like to enjoy . . . I like being
    with people you see, I like being social, I like having a laugh and stuff like that.
    I don't like sitting on my own with my thoughts, d'you understand me? . . . I like
    being with people. That's it.

For this individual, it is quite clear that the activity was of little interest in itself. However, he joined and regularly attended a golf programme on the basis of the social opportunities it provided. Within his description is a sense that this form of social involvement provided a focus for his thoughts that was preferable to spending time on his own.

A social orientation was very common among many participants who valued the opportunity to meet and make new friends through sport and exercise. When asked about his experience of being a member of a sport group, one participant replied:

It's a good social activity to be with them. It's a good time, to be with them. And you can learn by other people, what they've done as well I think, you can talk about it, you know. They'll probably ask, the other person, how you felt, and I think that's how you learn . . . it's a good atmosphere . . . It's different when you're not with a group as well isn't it? You get cut off a little bit don't you? I mean the atmosphere's not there so much, know what I mean?

This sense of social 'atmosphere' or occasion was something that we observed during group-based sports activities as the following excerpt from our field notes illustrates:

There seemed to be no interpersonal problems whatsoever. In fact, the group members were hugely generous and supportive of each other. One example was when William hit the ball off the tee ninety degrees into the rough. Immediately, Harry shouted out 'You can have that again.' Ronnie agreed, 'Yeah, he *can* have it again!' Similarly, on Harry holing out, Ronnie walked over and offered a 'fist handshake' and verbal congratulations. (David, 9 July)

A sense of support and consideration towards each other was also characteristic of these relationship stories and evident in many of the group activity sessions. One participant explicitly described the support he gained through the various sport and exercise groups he attended:

Well I'm sort of supported. I feel supported with other people there, yeah. It's people that I know mainly, especially like with the football team, it's people that I never knew before but I got friendly with – made good friends – and we all just participated in sport.

Often mutual support and consideration was unexpressed in verbal form during interviews being, instead, something that we observed enacted or unfolding within the dynamics of a group. As such, 'miniature' stories of consideration and generosity were not uncommon within day-to-day exchanges between group members. One example of this kind of relational orientation is demonstrated in the following excerpts from our field notes which, while referring to the same event, we both observed and recorded independently:

> Prior to the round, Richard had offered Chris a roll-up cigarette. Chris had replied 'Are you sure? Thanks very much' with an air of pleasant surprise that suggested perhaps it was not common for cigarettes to actually be offered round. On the sixth tee, Chris returned the generosity by asking whether Richard or I would like a cigarette. (David, 16 July)
>
> There is a gentleness and mutual respect between the group members. Typical of this are simple things like offering someone a cigarette ... Richard offered Chris a cigarette and Chris humbly looked and asked if Richard was sure. He asked in such a way that he gave away from his question that he took nothing for granted, that Richard didn't have to offer, it wasn't expected. (Kitrina, 16 July)

The importance of relationships is emphasised by Repper and Perkins (2003) as being central to fostering and maintaining hope during the recovery process. They point out that while professionals do not hold the key to recovery, professionals *do* have a role to play in facilitating and supporting relationships with others. We have seen how sport and physical activity can provide an environment in which these kinds of relationships can be initiated, nurtured and developed. Repper and Perkins (2003, p. 55) observe how 'in mental health services there is a tendency to regard relationships as a "one-way street" ... (when) meaningful relationships are as much about giving as receiving ... To reciprocate and help others makes one feel valued and worthwhile.' It was these kinds of relationships which participants spoke of and enacted through their sport and physical activity involvement.

Action, achievement and relationship stories and recovery

In chapter 1, we noted seven core themes in recovery, identified by people who have experienced mental health difficulties. These themes specify the need to:

(1) rebuild social roles and relationships;
(2) develop meaning and purpose in one's life;
(3) recreate a positive sense of self and identity;
(4) change one's attitudes, values and goals;
(5) enact, acquire and demonstrate ability;
(6) pursue personal interests, hopes, and aspirations;
(7) develop and maintain a sense of hopefulness about one's future.

Through exploring here three types of stories told by the participants in our research, we hope that the ways which physical activity and sport can contribute to these seven themes are beginning to become apparent. In the remainder of the chapter, we would like to explore the ways in which the kinds of narrative processes we have described can contribute to recovery.

Illness, time and recovery

Kathy Charmaz (1991) describes a change in a woman who became chronically ill in the following terms: 'Before she became ill, she had worked towards future goals. Afterwards, she sought valued moments and good days in the present' (p. 3). Participants' stories of sport and exercise have much in common with this description as, when they talked about activity, their stories were almost exclusively focused on the *present* – the here and now – and on valued moments and good experiences within the present. We think that a present-focus – as opposed to a focus on the past or distant future – is important in recovery terms because signifies a departure from restitution stories which, Sparkes and Smith (2003) suggest, are oriented towards reinstating *the past in the future*, a future in which wellness is expected to return. According to these authors, this is problematic because experiencing time in this way 'connects the individual to notions of a restored and entrenched self that has its reference point firmly in the past, all of which makes it difficult to develop different senses of self and explore alternative identities in the present' (p. 315).

By telling action, achievement and relationship stories in which they *kept busy* and *used time* in the present, participants immersed themselves in life *as it happened* and avoided living the script of potentially problematic future- or past-oriented stories. In so doing, each participant was able, as Charmaz (1991) describes, to locate their sense of self in a real and authentic present, rather than some previous remembered past or some hoped-for but distant future. Significantly, this real and authentic present became available for narration through personal and embodied involvement in sport and physical activity.

Self, meaning and recovery

Brendan Stone (2006) has identified three interrelated themes in published stories of mental illness: (i) a suspension from the social realm; (ii) a loss of speech which removes a person from the world of discourse and action; (iii) a radical disruption to sense of identity and the impression that selfhood is under threat. Narrative processes, he suggests, have the potential to help tackle these challenges. By storying one's experiences in the first person 'I', 'a self, or a sense of selfhood, is established which enables the speaker to look outside herself from that position' in a way that acts 'as a counterweight to the internalizing energies of psychosis' (Stone, 2006, p. 47). This process is demonstrated in the participants' stories of sport and physical activity which are invariably told in the first person – this simple act is a first step in establishing a sense of self which references one's own embodied experience. Additionally, the presence of *talk* – in the form of action, achievement and relationship stories – provides evidence of a reconnection with the social realm and re-engagement with shared discourse and action. In short, *doing* and *talking* signify two levels of involvement and interaction with the social world. Finally, the presence of relationship stories point towards awareness of interpersonal dimensions which contrast with the overriding self-focus which Stone (2006) observes in narratives of mental distress.

According to Baldwin (2005), an important component of therapeutic interventions for people with mental health problems is the opportunity to launch and maintain personal stories which reinstate a sense of meaning, identity and coherence in a person's life. In this regard, therapeutic initiatives should 'open space for persons to re-author or constitute themselves, each other and their relationships according to alternative stories or knowledges' (White & Epston, 1990, p. 75). By doing so, McLeod (1997) suggests, individuals have the opportunity to re-story their lives by creating and sharing personal stories which 'make sense' and are meaningful in the context of both their experience and the meta-narrative/s in which they are immersed. It is from this perspective, as Michele Crossley (2000, p. 21) observes, that the experience of self can be understood as taking 'on meaning only through specific linguistic, historical structures'. Put another way, without reference to biography, culture and language (i.e. talk, communication and stories), a sense of self can be neither developed nor maintained. Thus, as Crossley suggests, it is through narrative means that we define who we are, who we were and where we may be in the future. It is on this basis that the processes involved in creating and sharing the action, achievement and relationship stories enabled participants to re-story their lives in ways that supported the exploration of alternative identities and selves.

Adventure and recovery

It has been suggested that people require narrative resources – perhaps in the form of *adventures* – in order to re-story their lives (Scheibe, 1986). 'Adventure' experiences can trigger – or form the foundations of – new or alternative life stories. The *Concise Oxford English Dictionary* defines *adventure* as 'an unusual, exciting, or daring experience' and we think this definition captures the place sport and physical activity holds in some people's lives. According to McLeod (1997, p. 43):

> Different people may draw upon different sources of adventure. However, each type of adventure gives the person a ready supply of stories through which to create an identity both in the form of an ongoing self-narrative but also a narrative that is shared with, and co-constructed with, other people. Adventurous activities also furnish a reference group of others willing to listen to these stories, as in groups of anglers 'swapping' tales of fish caught and fish that got away.

As McLeod observes, 'adventure' means different things to different people – football, for example, may constitute an adventure for one but not for another. However, among the participants in our research, most were able to find a form of sport or physical activity which they seemed to experience as 'adventure' and which provided concrete, embodied experiences to talk about (in the form of action and achievement stories), alongside day-to-day opportunities to share these stories with others (in the form of relationship stories). As such, sport and physical activity were simultaneously a shared experience to *talk about* and an opportunity *to talk*. From the perspective of recovery, these opportunities are important because, as Chadwick (2009) points out:

even extremely withdrawn people value being treated not as 'mental patients' . . . they need to be spoken to at times not as patients but as persons. It is therefore useful to talk to them about ordinary things like local football or fashion news, things in the paper generally and matters other than medication, medication effects, cognitive and psycho-dynamic distortions and their general mental state. They enjoy ordinary everyday chatter; it is a change from the 'illness talk' that often surrounds them. That in itself only keeps reminding them over and over again of their position. They can do without it because first and foremost they are people-in-the-world and only secondarily patients or residents-in-care. (p. 133)

Key points

- This chapter has highlighted a second way in which involvement in sport or physical activity can contribute to recovery in the context of mental illness, namely through providing the narrative resources which enable individuals to create and share positive personal stories which differ markedly from the dominant and more negative meta-narrative of mental illness.
- Through telling present-focused stories of their sport and exercise experiences – built around the notions of action, achievement and relationships – individuals have the opportunity to re-story their lives through reconstructing or sustaining a more positive, hopeful and meaningful identity and sense of self independent of mental health culture.
- Activities which are experienced by an individual as an 'adventure' are likely to be effective in stimulating and supporting new and alternative life stories.
- While *doing* an activity is important, it is not necessarily *sufficient*: the processes involved in creating and sharing *stories* of one's experience are also important from the perspective of recovery.

Implications

- Alongside participation, there is much to be gained in recovery terms when opportunities are made available for individuals to communicate and interact with others about their sport or activity experiences. We therefore suggest that those who organise sport and physical activity initiatives in mental health settings consider ways to facilitate and support verbal interaction during and following sessions. Possible strategies include reciprocal coaching, talk-and-walk sessions, scheduling shared refreshment breaks, scheduling a social 'get together' after the activity, and planning periodic social get-togethers to share photographs/videos/memories of the group's activities.
- Action stories depend upon an individual *doing* and being *involved* or *immersed* in the activity. These stories may be promoted and facilitated through offering sport or physical activity opportunities which capture an individual's interest and are experienced as an 'adventure'. Choosing unusual or novel forms of sport/activity, travelling to different locations, changing the activity periodically, customising the

activity in unusual ways, including music, trying outdoor activity or dance are all strategies which have the potential to preserve a degree of surprise or novelty which is likely to stimulate and support the creation and sharing of new action stories.

■ Achievement stories depend upon a personal sense of *success* or *accomplishment*. Performance outcomes are the dominant way in which achievement is typically measured in sport or physical activity, but this approach can bring problems, as we discuss in chapter 7. While success in a tournament, competition or race might lead to a sense of achievement, failure often has the opposite effect. We recommend that if performance outcomes are employed, an individual-specific focus is adopted which focuses on personal progression and milestones. Additionally, a sense of achievement can arise from process factors such as mastery of new tasks, contributing to others' development or enjoyment of an activity, meeting new people, visiting new places or completing a programme of activity.

■ Relationship stories depend on involvement with and consideration of others. Group activities are most likely to allow for this opportunity, but individual activities (such as running, gym training, walking the dog, swimming) can also be effective if individuals have opportunities (during or following the activity) to share their experience (e.g. through club membership, through a drink in the leisure centre café afterwards, through chatting with other dog walkers). A sport coach or exercise leader who values relationships as a worthwhile outcome of participation can do much to encourage similar values among group members.

Physical activity as a stepping stone in recovery

6

It's not made me into a different person. I'm still Mark ... but I feel a bit more energised, a bit more with it than I did before I started.

Mark

In this chapter we explore the ways in which participation in physical activity or sport can act as a *stepping stone* or *vehicle* in the process of recovering from mental health problems. As the words of one participant (quoted above) suggest, participation in sport or physical activity is not always a life-changing event of great personal significance. Instead, it is an activity which provides some kind of personally meaningful *outcome* which is considered by the individual to be beneficial. Using activity as a 'stepping stone' is a third way in which physical activity and sport can contribute to recovery, contrasting with those we described in chapters 4 and 5 where the benefits of participation are more to do with the *process* of participation than the outcomes.

A brief case study

One participant in our research, named Mark, provides a good example of an individual who 'uses' physical activity and sport as a stepping stone or vehicle for other things (see Carless & Douglas, 2008b). In contrast to Ben (see chapter 4), Mark displayed no real signs of sport or exercise being important aspects of his identity, his sense of who is as a person. Although Mark described a history of sport participation as a young man, his involvement ended when he left school. It wasn't until 18 years later that Mark engaged again in sport or exercise and, tellingly, he described his activity as 'starting afresh'. Mark displayed no biographical markers linking his sense of self to sport: he did not wear sports clothing or talk about watching sporting events and he owned no sporting equipment or memorabilia. Likewise, Mark rarely engaged in sport-related conversations with other service users or mental health professionals. For Mark, rather than being a central, intrinsic component of his identity and sense of self, physical activity and sport seem to be meaningful only to the extent that they bring about extrinsic *consequences* or *outcomes* which hold value and meaning within the broader context of his life. Two consequences, we suggest, were particularly important to Mark.

First, Mark valued being able to take part in an activity which kept him busy and filled his time. As we discussed in chapter 5, other research (Raine *et al.*, 2002; Faulkner & Biddle, 2004; McDevitt *et al.*, 2006) has also identified keeping busy as a positive consequence of sport and exercise participation in mental health settings. For Mark, keeping busy took on a further dimension because he believed that by keeping busy with sport and exercise he was making positive use of his time, that he was engaging in a worthwhile activity. That sport and exercise are considered worthwhile by Mark relates to a second consequence of participation: perceived improvements in fitness. Thus, Mark attributed perceived fitness improvements to his sport and exercise participation, and these improvements better equipped him to meet the physical demands of his chosen vocational activities which were gardening and woodwork. Generalised fitness improvements allowed Mark to more fully engage in activities such as gardening and woodwork, and it is these activities which hold personal meaning and value. It is these activities we think which, to use Patricia Deegan's (1996) terminology, coincide with the person Mark would like to become and, perhaps, provide him with a reason to 'say yes to life'. It is in this sense that, as Pamela Raine and colleagues (2002) have also identified, physical activity and sport have served as a stepping stone in his journey towards recovery.

In what follows, we would like to explore in turn seven outcomes which other participants described as arising from their physical activity and sport participation. These outcomes are:

- symptom alleviation
- positive affect or mood
- cognitive improvement
- relaxation and stress relief
- keeping busy and filling time
- social connectedness
- physical fitness and body weight.

Symptom alleviation

As we discussed in chapter 1, a good deal of physical activity and mental health research has focused primarily or exclusively on the extent to which physical activity alleviates the symptoms of mental illness. Notwithstanding the problems we have identified with this focus, some participants in our research described benefits in these terms. Considering his participation in a sport group one individual, for example, said: 'I'm surprised that I've enjoyed it this much actually. I'm not getting as many, I don't know what it is, side effects or symptoms or whatever.' In a similarly general manner another described how 'It [exercise] has helped my mental health problem. I realise I've got a mental health problem and, uh, it's coming to terms with it. But, doing the exercise, that helps I think, it's a benefit.' The following excerpts taken from interviews with three individuals provide some further insights.

Kitrina: Do you think playing golf particularly helps your mental health problems?
[Pause] Uh. I wouldn't say it gets rid of it but it does, uh, say it's like a battery then, it's like a battery. It lasts for so long, then.

Sarah [during a focus group]: Shaun, just going back to your poem, one line that says football stops you thinking about your bad thoughts, something like that, can you say a little bit more about what you meant perhaps by that?
Just in a sense that my mind's occupied. I think other things – I don't really think about bad things that I might think about if I wasn't doing something.
Sarah: Is it doing something specifically like sport or does that happen with anything?
It can happen with other things but I think sport is such an active thing it tends to have that effect on me. When I'm watching it as well you know, when I go to watch it.

Kitrina: So particularly with coping with your illness, does it [golf] help there at all?
[Pause] In a small part, yeah.
Kitrina: Can you describe the small part that it might help?
Um, it gets you [pause] it gets your mind on another track, while it's on.
Kitrina: But then your mind would go back into the track after or not?
Not permanently. It doesn't have a permanent effect.
Kitrina: Are there other things that have a similar effect? [pause] 'Cause you do painting as well...
I paint, that has a permanent effect. That shoots trouble for good ... When you've got mental health problems, just distraction alone is not really the answer. You need more. You need to shoot the problems.
Kitrina: Uh huh [pause]. And golf hasn't shot any of your problems?
Not really. It takes your mind off temporarily while it's going on but when it finishes, back to the norm.

While some individuals, as these examples suggest, described temporary symptomatic relief, it was rare for any individual to explicitly state in an unambiguous manner that activity alleviated the symptoms of illness. Other individuals felt that, while their activity provided benefits, symptom alleviation was not really one of them. For us, these excerpts reveal some of the problems behind any claims for a role for physical activity in alleviating the symptoms of mental health problems. As we see it, there are two possible reasons for a general absence of instances when individuals stated in a concrete fashion that activity helped their mental illness.

First, given the complexity and severity of the mental health problems of the participants in our research (and, therefore, their recovery needs), it is unreasonable to expect *any* single intervention to provide 'the answer'. Second, on analysing and reflecting upon our interview data we were struck by a general *absence* of talk and conversation about the symptoms of mental illness. This isn't to say that participants were not experiencing symptoms, but rather that symptoms were not a common focus of conversation. In other words, in the context of sport and physical activity sessions, conversation rarely revolved around mental health problems. We think the absence of this kind of talk was a *strength* of the activity groups (as we discussed in chapters 4 and 5). Thus, it was generally only when we – as researchers – explicitly asked about symptoms or illness that participants made reference to this issue. This can be seen in the three preceding excerpts. When participants responded to a question relating to symptom alleviation, responses ranged from a resounding 'yes' to a clear 'no' with pretty much every gradation in between. Our interpretation of these responses is that physical activity and sport *can* help alleviate the symptoms of mental distress for *some* people *some* of the time, but that a stable, universal relationship does not exist. It is through other channels that sport or activity is more likely to contribute to recovery, such as those described in chapters 4 and 5 and in the remainder of this chapter.

Positive affect

Researchers have documented the occurrence of positive affect (i.e. positive feelings, mood or emotions) through participation in various forms of physical activity and this response have been observed among people who are experiencing a mental health problem (such as depression, anxiety or schizophrenia) as well as among individuals with no diagnosed mental health problem. Positive affect was described by participants in our research in a number of ways and as stemming from diverse forms of activity. Some described it in terms which relate to a sense of increased optimism, enjoyment or excitement. In the words of two individuals:

David: Do you think football makes you a different person in any way?
I think it's helped me a lot. I feel a lot more positive in myself. I've just been trying to organise this football league thing and stuff has been sort of quite beneficial to me really. Something to think about and something I get quite excited about to some extent.

When I'm exercising it makes you feel up for it. It makes you feel good about yourself as well. When I'm actually exercising no matter what I feel like I don't feel depressed or anything. I always feel good no matter when I'm exercising – just makes me feel good.

Others described activity as providing some kinds of mood improvement:

When I was low I was in, I had, like, different mood levels. And, you know, the medication I was on that would like alternate the moods I was in. So when I took that it gave me a lift. But when I was doing exercises it was similar to that like, it gave me a lift similar to what I was on with the medication.

Sometimes you can feel better than other days. If you had a bit of a bad day and felt a bit low – run and you feel great again ... One minute you're depressed – you go out for a run and you're feeling good again.

At times, participants' descriptions communicated a generalised sense of a positive psychological response such as Mark's statement that 'I feel healthier, more refreshed when I'm playing football.' Inherent in this remark is the suggestion of a link between feeling good *psychologically* and feeling good *physically*. This link is developed in one individual's description of running:

> I suppose it makes you face the problem head on. It makes you feel as though it's not that bad in the first place. There's nothing really to worry about. Whether it's the endorphins it releases in the system. I think it makes you feel positive about yourself. Because you're getting fit and exercising, what you're doing there is things that are positive and it's making you think positive and feel positive as well.

Of note in these excerpts is a deviation away from describing the psychological effects of activity in terms of removing negative experiences from one's life, as is the case in symptom alleviation terms. In other words, participants commonly described activity not in terms of what it *took away* from their life, but what it *added to* their life. In this sense, sport and activity are described in positive terms as ways to enhance one's existence in ways that, for the most part, *anybody* might appreciate regardless of whether or not they were experiencing a diagnosed mental health problem. Understanding participants' descriptions of positive affect as, to some extent, independent of mental illness allows a connection to be made between users of mental health services and the general population. In our experience positive psychological responses to physical activity should not be expected to differ between those who are experiencing mental illness and those who are not: the psychological differences will be *within* each group rather than *between* each group. The most likely difference between these two populations is the heightened significance and value positive responses may hold for individuals with a mental illness who may have fewer alternative avenues in their lives (e.g. due to lack of employment, inadequate housing, poverty, restricted social networks, stigmatisation) through which to feel good about themselves.

Cognitive improvement

Several participants described what might be generally considered improved cognitive function through involvement in a particular form of sport or physical activity. This benefit was described in terms of improved concentration, clear thinking or greater focus through having something specifically to think about. For example, in the words of two individuals:

David: What sort of things are important in your general well-being?
Well, being able to concentrate on what you're doing at a specific time. Talking to someone and listen to them as well – what they are actually saying.
David: Right. So the exercise helps with that?
Yeah, 'cause you're concentrating. It helps you to think better, it helps you to concentrate better on what you're doing, when you're actually doing the exercise, the football, badminton. With badminton you have to use hand-eye co-ordination to bring your racket back and follow through the stroke. So I mean that's a benefit, 'cause you're concentrating.

You think more when you're running. I think. You can work things out. Things that are bad don't seem that bad anyway ... everything becomes more clear, you, yeah, everything becomes more clear, like. You can think more, you can solve your problems a bit, like. I think more running than what I do in bed at night really.

Some participants described these kinds of improvements as counteracting what they experienced as side effects of antipsychotic medication which, in one individual's terms, made him feel 'fuzzy'. In these kinds of descriptions, taking part in exercise allowed them to regain a sense of mental sharpness or focus. Other descriptions struck us as being more about a personal need – which we all share – to have something to do and therefore something to think *about*. This orientation seems less about distracting oneself *away from* a problem, and more to do with having something positive to focus one's thoughts *towards*. For some individuals, some form of sport or physical activity was sufficient to provide this focus.

Relaxation and stress relief

In the straightforward but revealing words of one participant, when taking part in sport (in this case, golf) 'I just feel quite relaxed like, or [pause] OK, kind of normal.' Besides being one form of 'normal' leisure activity which can connect a person with mainstream culture and society outside mental health (as we discussed in chapter 5), certain forms of sport or exercise were experienced by some participants as providing a sense of relaxation or stress relief. This is demonstrated in the following excerpts:

I don't intend to be like, very serious with it, it's just quite enjoyable, gets rid of some stress ... physical exercise can un-stress me.
David: Right, so if you've got hassles from other things?
Yeah, yeah, got [pause], oh, hassles like certain situations when I might feel panicky, get a panic attack ... all sports seem to help with that.

Kitrina: Do you think that golf is good for your mind, the way you think about things?
Yeah, it relaxes you, like. You can switch off I think. If you was worried about something, I'm trying to think, squash is a similar game I think, if you were really anxious and, anxiety, you're really in an annoying mood or you feel really upset about something, I think when you play squash, you come out of that door and you feel totally different like ... All your frustration's gone like. It's like a balloon, let it out of the balloon like, it's like all the anxiety and that, frustration, is out.

When you're exercising on your own it's sort of, sort of, tranquillity really in a way. A strange sense of tranquillity I suppose. Makes you feel at one.

I felt keen, you know, cause I felt it was good time out and, you know, it's not as if I'm playing a hectic sport, it [golf] is pretty relaxed ... it looked a very relaxed style sport – that's the beauty of it. Plus it's out and about.

There is a good deal of variability among those individuals who identified stress relief or relaxation as an outcome of their physical activity, both in terms of what aspect of the experience it was that *provided* the relief and what the relief was *from*. At times, some participants explicitly connected the sense of relaxation or stress relief to specific mental health problems. More often, however, the sense of stress relief was related to everyday situations and issues which most people are likely to experience from time to time (e.g. financial problems, bereavement, relationship difficulties).

It is more difficult to identify which aspects of sport or exercise provided a sense of relaxation or stress relief. In our research, a golf activity group was frequently cited as being experienced as relaxing by group members and, given the nature of the game when played as a leisure activity (outdoors in a pleasant environment, relatively slow pace, opportunities for social interaction), this is not surprising. One participant described the process of playing as related to relaxation:

> Last week was lovely 'cause I felt quite relaxed. Although I didn't hit the ball very well, I found it relaxing … When I got the swing going I started to enjoy it and find it relaxing like as well … it's scenery, yeah. When you see a ball go down a fairway you think 'Whoa! That looks good doesn't it!' You just feel good about it. I think you feel relaxed because you've hit the ball quite well.

In this description there is a sense that, once again, an array of factors contributed to creating an experience that is interpreted in positive terms. While this individual suggests that adverse performance outcomes (i.e. not hitting the ball very well) did not reduce his relaxation, he suggests several factors that *were* important: getting 'the swing going', the scenery, seeing the ball travel down a fairway and feeling good about a shot. In this light, rather than a singular quality or 'mechanism' resulting in feelings of relaxation, we see the holistic 'social experience' inherent in a good physical activity or sport session as providing relief from day-to-day stresses and promoting feelings of relaxation. It is, however, important to bear in mind that not *all* physical activity and sport sessions are likely to result in this kind of outcome (see Part III).

Keeping busy and filling time

We were surprised how often participants cite keeping busy and filling time as beneficial 'outcomes' of sport or physical activity participation. Perhaps when the typical social context of mental illness is considered, this should not be surprising. As we noted in chapters 1 and 5, survivor stories of mental illness frequently describe periods of boredom, monotony, of having nothing to do. For most of us, prolonged or continued 'empty time' is a negative experience. Sometimes, the desire to fill or make use of one's time serves as a motivator for becoming involved in sport or physical activity, as the following excerpt reveals:

David: *What was it that made you think of starting the exercise again?*
I realised that I could use my time better … That's important I think – to actually be able to use your time properly … I've got the time to exercise so I use it.

This individual described how some of the positive feelings he experiences stem from the belief that, by exercising, he is making good use of his time. As he put it, when talking about his participation in a five-a-side football group:

> I enjoy it, have a sense of satisfaction that I actually played because I was doing something with my time. That's important I think – to actually be able to use your

time properly . . . I know I haven't wasted my time, I've used my time constructively doing something that'll do me good.

David: *Are there any things that you find make it difficult for you to go and exercise? Anything that gets in the way?*

No, not at the moment. I've got the time to exercise so I use it . . . I'm not gonna slack and give it up 'cause I realise using my time better is important.

It is through considering the social context of mental illness, and in particular the lack of alternative activities that many users of mental health services describe, that the personal importance or significance of keeping busy with an activity that is perceived 'worthwhile' is best appreciated. Referring to his involvement in a sport group, one individual stated simply: 'It's something to get me out of bed, get me out of bed that morning.' We suggest that this simple outcome can be profoundly important if a person has little else scheduled for her or his day. Having something 'on the agenda' is, after all, important for us all.

Social connectedness

While it was unusual for any individual in our research to specifically cite social connectedness as a motive for joining a physical activity or sport group, an appreciation for the importance and value of being with others and doing things with others was often evident. As we discussed in chapter 5, building relationships with others through shared experiences and opportunities to talk about those experiences is an important component of many people's activity experiences. For some, social connectedness may be the most important motivator and outcome of participation (see chapter 8). This outcome can be important, we suggest, at more or less *any* point in the recovery process and for a person experiencing anything from 'mild' psychological difficulties through to, potentially, hospitalisation during an acute psychotic episode. For example, one exercise leader described his first impressions of a young man who was hospitalised during an acute episode of schizophrenia:

Shaun was one of the first people I met when I started at Brentree Hospital about three years ago. He was on a secure unit, wouldn't say boo to a goose, even in that secure unit he would keep himself to himself, wouldn't say anything, but when I asked if he wanted a game of football he'd go out and play a game. That was the only way he expressed himself, that was the only thing he would do and interact with anyone. I wouldn't say too much – or anything at all – head down, like this *[mimes looking at the ground and avoiding eye contact]* like that, just kicking a ball, doing his keep-ups.

Another individual described the role that activity groups played while he was in hospital:

I started going to gym and went to OT and then I started going swimming – that was it then. It wasn't so bad then. I was actually on the road to recovery . . . I started talking and got out of my shell. It was important to like to talk to people – communicate with people. So all that was on my own part really, I done it myself, started to talk to people myself. Once I started talking to people it gave me more confidence.

Often, social connectedness continues to be important to individuals even when they are no longer experiencing acute difficulties. After leaving hospital Colin, for instance, moved into supported accommodation and attended a rehabilitation day centre which served as the base for, among other things, his ongoing sport and physical activities. As he put it:

I'm sort of supported, I feel supported with other people there, it's people that I know mainly. Especially like with the football team, it's people that I never knew before but I got friendly with, made good friends, and we all just participated in sport.

Other participants described the benefits of some kind of social connectedness through activity simply as a 'natural' and 'enjoyable' way to be. For these individuals, for an activity to be worthwhile it need not achieve anything more than providing an opportunity or avenue through which they could be with and interact with others.

Physical fitness and body weight

Overweight and obesity is often cited as a significant health concern in Western societies (e.g. Department of Health, 2004) and regular participation in physical activity is routinely promoted on the basis of its role as a weight management strategy. People who are experiencing mental health difficulties are not immune to the risk of obesity and its effects on long-term health and, common sense would suggest, are likely to be faced with very much the same challenges as people without a diagnosed mental health problem. The risk of obesity is further increased among individuals who are taking antipsychotic medication because a common side effect of such medication is significant weight gain (Allison *et al.*, 1999; Green *et al.*, 2000). Paradoxically, there is also a risk for some people of *weight loss* as a consequence of or co-occuring factor in depression. While body weight issues have not been an explicit focus of our research, they have inevitably cropped up as issues which are related to physical activity and sport participation. We feel it is relevant to briefly explore participants' accounts of weight gain and weight loss in relation to their physical activity.

Ben's experiences (see chapter 4) provide an illustration of the possibility of significant weight gain alongside the experience of psychotic illness, in this case schizophrenia. During the acute phases of illness, Ben experienced significant weight gain which he attributed to a combination of the side effects of the antipsychotic medications he had been prescribed and an extended period of physical inactivity. As we discussed in chapter 4, Ben was troubled by his body weight partly because it impeded his running performance and his ability to participate in longer races. In response to a question about whether he was setting targets to improve during his running training, Ben said:

Well, at the moment I'm just doing it. I'm not really timing myself or anything. I'm just doing it to get my weight off you know what I mean. I'm just hoping that it'll help, contribute to some weight loss at the moment. But I suppose when I get my weight off I'll time myself down and try and do it quicker.

For Ben, it seemed that it was more the case that his increased body weight got in the way of his competitive race plans and inhibited his improvement as a runner. He described his dietary programme as the primary way in which he tried to reduce his weight to allow him to run better, but did not seem to take part in running for the outcome of weight loss.

Colin, in contrast, described part of his motivation for activity as relating to the desired outcome of weight loss. He had complex experiences of weight change through his changing experiences of illness, medication and physical activity. The following excerpt provides a sense of this changing terrain:

I knew I'd lost weight [in hospital] but I didn't realise how it could have been quite serious really ... Partly because of the depression that I was in – the mental state I was in – I didn't have a lot of food really ... I lost a lot of weight then. I didn't like the food in the hospital, didn't have a lot of food that I would like at home ... I had a meal but I didn't really have a lot of food that I should have had. And then when I left hospital I started to drink. After that I think that's why I put my weight on, like ... I wish I was that weight now, not *so* thin, but I must have been about $11\frac{1}{2}$ to 12 stone then. It's not so bad now, although I got a weight now, 'cause I'm tall it doesn't really show so much does it? But I feel myself that it does. I've got a guilty conscience about my weight and I've always told the doctor that I want to lose weight anyway.

In the first half of this excerpt an important issue is voiced relating to the potentially adverse contribution of physical activity to the health and well-being of a person experiencing weight loss alongside depression. There is a body of evidence which highlights the ways in which 'excessive' levels of exercise, for some people and at certain times, can contribute to psychological health difficulties such as eating disorders (see, for example, Zanker & Gard, 2008). At this point in his history, high levels of exercise participation are likely to have been a further threat to Colin's physical health and well-being. Having left hospital, however, his experiences changed dramatically to the point that he experienced significant weight gain. It was at this time that physical activity became a conscious component of Colin's weight management strategy. In this instance, as for some others who were experiencing weight gain as a side effect of medication, physical activity participation came to be motivated – in part at least – on the basis of its potential to help reduce body weight through increasing daily energy uptake and therefore calorific consumption. It is this outcome, for some people, which forms the basis of their ongoing participation.

For some, the potential of exercise to improve physical fitness is an important outcome and motivator for involvement. Mark's experiences provide an illustration of the way this process can be important for some individuals. In response to a question about what benefits he perceived from his sport and exercise participation, Mark replied:

Well it helps me build up my strength for digging the weeds in the allotment. Just general digging the ground cause I've got the strength to do it much easier than when I felt weak. It's made me feel stronger, capable of doing the gardening – it gives you satisfaction that way . . . I'm a bit fitter than I used to be. Like doing the woodwork – I can saw pieces of wood easier. I feel stronger in myself. It's got me a bit fitter.

While at first glance these benefits might appear minor or unimportant, for a person like Mark we suggest that they can be quite significant and highly valued. This was particularly the case because Mark's vocational aspirations were focused on obtaining work as a gardener. In the context of the poor fitness he described during earlier phases of his illness (which he associated with very low levels of physical activity), these fitness improvements were personally meaningful and necessary if he was to be physically capable of gardening work.

A tangled web

More than ten years ago, Ken Fox (1999) wrote that the mental health effects of exercise should be understood as a *horses for courses* phenomenon. When the outcomes of physical activity in mental health contexts are examined in the way we have in this chapter – through seeking to identify and understand themes within participants' accounts – this is a good analogy. It seems to us, too, that a complex relationship exists between the characteristics and needs of the individual, the type of sport or physical activity in question, and the particular combination of outcomes that arise through participation. In short, the precise effects are individual-specific (Carless & Faulkner, 2003; Faulkner & Carless, 2006).

More often than not, perhaps, any one individual will experience a 'cocktail' of benefits which may be difficult to untangle. Many of the participants in our research described – what seems to us at least – a 'tangled web' of factors which affected their journey towards recovery. For example, Sarah (a physiotherapist at a vocational rehabilitation day centre for people with severe and enduring mental health problems) made the following remarks about Shaun, a young man diagnosed with schizophrenia:

> Three years ago when he came he would pace the car park. He was up-down, up-down for ages. He would never ever make eye contact. He would always look *[mimes looking away]* like that whenever he spoke to you. I mean he's just, just a different person really . . . It's difficult to work out how much is the actual exercise that's helping him and how much it's the, sort of, with the projects. But I mean this five-a-side league thing that's only very recent, that's the last six months or so.

For some individuals, the point was that sport or exercise provided a range of benefits and there was no particular need to identify what, exactly, had helped them. The following excerpt provides an example of this:

David: Are there certain things that you can put your finger on and say 'I really feel better about that particular thing' or this particular way?

Well, it's better all the way round really. It makes you, I mean, you lose weight, you feel fitter, you feel better, you feel you can tackle any task and you, um, you feel you can take on anything really. You feel that confident . . . You're walking down a road you feel, you think, yeah, you're up for it – you're ready. I'm ready to tackle the day, you know.

We see these various outcomes of physical activity or sport as related to personal *meaning* – whether a particular outcome is valuable to the individual depends on the subjective processes through which that person construes meaning in his or her life. It is quite feasible, or even likely, that each of the outcomes discussed above, while being personally meaningful to one person, might hold no value to another. For example, although Mark identified 'keeping busy' and improving fitness as meaningful outcomes and motives for activity, these were of little interest to Ronnie who said his primary goal for taking part in an activity group was social connectedness. Therefore, it is not the case that *any* outcome will be experienced as beneficial (or, for that matter, experienced at all) by *any* individual but rather that the degree to which an outcome is beneficial will depend on that individual's history, interests, aspirations and hopes. Simply put, should an outcome 'fit' or 'match' with any of these factors then it is likely it will be experienced as beneficial. Appreciating the individual ways in which the outcomes of activity may be experienced points to the need to consider carefully each person's needs, goals and preferences when it comes to offering sport and physical activity opportunities in mental health contexts.

Key points

- Some people experience particular *outcomes* of physical activity or sport participation which motivate their continued involvement. Evident in these descriptions are portrayals of participation as a *vehicle* or *stepping stone* which makes it possible for an individual to – in some way – move on in life. This orientation is entirely consistent with the ethos of exercise and health promotion initiatives which typically promote participation on the basis of extrinsic outcomes.
- Participants in our research have described a range of outcomes from sport and physical activity involvement which include symptom alleviation, positive affect or mood, cognitive improvements, relaxation and stress relief, keeping busy and filling time, social connectedness, physical fitness and body weight changes.
- This kind of extrinsic outcome-focused orientation is, however, just one part of a more complex picture. Often (as we discussed in chapters 4 and 5), a different type of story was told by participants which portrayed the *process* of sport and exercise as somehow integral to a person's life, holding meaning in terms of identity, sense of self and hopes for the future.
- We suggest that the ways physical activity and sport can act as a stepping stone depend upon the circumstances and aspirations of the individual. To provide outcomes which are experienced as personally meaningful – and hence beneficial – it is necessary to pay close attention to the history, needs, preferences and aspirations of each individual. It is not the case that a standardised 'prescription' of exercise will result in outcomes which are experienced as beneficial by all people.

Implications

- Understanding the distinct roles physical activity and sport play for different people can assist in the provision of personally meaningful physical activity and sport opportunities.
- Some people use sport and exercise in an instrumental fashion – as a vehicle or tool which indirectly equips them to pursue other activities which hold personal meaning and value. In this guise, participation is not for its own intrinsic sake but oriented towards achieving some kind of extrinsic benefit. Hence the appeal of physical activity and sport lies in its outcomes because these outcomes facilitate other personally relevant roles and activities. In addition to encouragement and practical assistance to support initial participation, these individuals are likely to benefit from education concerning the ways in which the outcomes of sport and physical activity participation (e.g. fitness, keeping busy, social connectedness) can help them move on.
- For a coach or practitioner who is passionate about sport or physical activity and enthusiastic to get others involved, the prospect of an individual who might use sport as a short-lived stepping stone to other things might be de-motivating. This orientation, however, should not diminish the potential importance of short-term activity sessions as the outcomes they provide may prove to be a critical and integral ingredient of an individual's recovery.
- From this perspective, little is lost when the individual ceases participation in an activity in order to commence something new. Cessation – when viewed in these terms – does not imply failure.

Part III

Practice and provision of physical activity and sport

7

The culture of physical activity and sport

Like the fish, it is so easy to be blind . . . to the all-pervading water in which one swims and the enormous (often 'too tiny to notice or mention') interchanges within it.

Peter Chadwick (2009, p. 120)

In some ways a chapter on the culture of sport and physical activity may seem out of place in a book about physical activity and mental health. As human beings, however, we exist in a social world and our lives are inevitably influenced by the culture in which we live. In the same way as fish are immersed in water – their lives profoundly shaped by its (we imagine) unnoticed presence – so too are we immersed in, shaped by yet often blind to, our own culture. If we are to understand the ways physical activity and sport may affect mental health, it is necessary to consider and reflect upon the cultural contexts in which sport and physical activity take place. Because cultural factors influence the extent to which sport and physical activity is likely to be experienced as beneficial, a degree of cultural awareness will assist with the planning and provision of successful physical activity and sport opportunities. One way to raise this kind of awareness is to explore how culturally situated narratives influence physical activity and sport experiences.

To do this we try to step back and consider the 'landscape' of physical activity and sport to make explicit some key assumptions and values that are sometimes overlooked. One example is a widespread positive disposition towards sport and physical activity in contemporary Western culture – an almost 'evangelical zeal' regarding its benefits. It doesn't take many visits to big sporting events to realise how many people really enjoy sport, and the central role sport plays in many people's lives. Commonly, those who have positive, reinforcing and joyous memories in sport remain enthusiastic even when they stop playing. Many former performers go on to become coaches or administrators or take other leadership roles. As a result, there is a risk of a culture which sees the effects of sport and physical activity through rose-tinted spectacles which distort or suppress the sometimes damaging effects of involvement. If your sport experiences have been generally positive, and if you are enthusiastic and want to put back into an activity that has given you so much, it can be difficult to become aware of the kinds of problematic issues that cause other people to drop out of physical activity or sport, or not engage in the first place. It is these issues which we focus on in this chapter as a way of encouraging you to reflect on your own attitudes and expectations concerning physical activity and sport. This kind of reflective practice is important because the attitudes and expectations of coaches and exercise leaders inevitably influence the experiences of those who attend their sessions.

The physical activity landscape

From a quick look through the promotional literature of most health clubs – and even recent policy documents (see, for example, Department for Culture, Media and Sport, 2002, 2008) – it might appear that physical activity has only positive consequences. Diet and exercising don't just promise to help you lose weight, they promise to make you 'look good' and 'feel great' (Northcott, 2009). Going to the gym doesn't just increase strength and fitness, it promises to boost your confidence and 'sculpt the body you aspire to' (David Lloyd Leisure, 2009). The profusion of research into all aspects of exercise and health has meant that practitioners who work in exercise contexts are aware of the benefits of regular physical activity, and can say with confidence that it reduces the risk of premature death from cardiovascular disease, some cancers and type 2 diabetes and can improve psychological well-being (Department of Health, 2004).

As a result of these benefits, the Chief Medical Officer (Department of Health, 2004, p. 3) recommends that adults should undertake:

- at least 30 minutes of physical activity five days a week which can be broken into smaller time segments;
- 45–60 minutes of moderate intensity physical activity per day in order to prevent obesity;
- activity in the form of lifestyle activities, structured exercise, sport or a combination of all three.

Practitioners now have established protocols and criteria with which to assess and monitor clients' fitness levels and the ability to prescribe activities which increase their flexibility, aerobic capacity, muscular strength and endurance. In short, health clubs, gyms, personal trainers and coaches know why physical activity is important for health and have the tools to help people become fitter and healthier.

With an emphasis on a healthier *body*, the drive for improved health exists, however, within a narrow biologically defined definition of what it is to be 'healthy' – no longer are rosy cheeks and a smiling face sufficient! Through the media, advertisements on television and in magazines, as well as through visits to the GP, health clubs, gyms and so on, we are all encouraged to 'police' our bodies more closely: to monitor and control our own body weight, blood pressure, cholesterol, alcohol consumption, time spent in the sun and so on. Those who fail to adopt the current health guidelines and engage in this kind of self-monitoring can easily come to be viewed as 'deviant'. As Shilling (2005, p. 160) notes, an 'increasing social cachet is attached to the slim body, and a growing prejudice aimed at those who do not achieve this body type'.

Conner and Armitage (2000, pp. 77–78) describe cultural messages and expectations about body weight as a 'prejudice' which:

> begins in childhood, with children preferring not to play with overweight peers and assigning negative adjectives to drawings of overweight individuals. In adulthood, overweight individuals tend to be rated as less attractive and athletic, but also less intelligent, hard working, successful and popular. They also face prejudice in relation to getting into college and getting good jobs ... Such negative views of the overweight individual appear to be particularly common in individualistic cultures where individuals are held to be responsible for their own fates.

By individualistic cultures, Conner and Armitage allude to those cultures where autonomy, independence and self-directedness are highly valued and are associated with strength (both physical and mental), while structural inequalities – which mitigate against healthy living for certain sections of society – are denied (Hayland, 1988). Consequently a fat, unfit body can come to be seen as a sign of a weak individual or an individual who has chosen not to have a slim, healthy body. Under such a lens the overweight or unfit person becomes a problem, not necessarily for the individual, but for a society preoccupied with a health agenda. Those who smoke, who are overweight, or who make other lifestyle choices which are deemed to be unhealthy are at an increased risk of stigma, moral indignation or hostility and even risk having future healthcare withheld or restricted (see Sparkes, 1997). In this climate, it is possible that any individual, regardless of their background, health status, age or ethnicity, will face a degree of shame or stigma if their body does not conform to the *ideal* image even if this image is unrealistic or unachievable.

Those who enter sport and physical activity environments as part of a mental health programme are not immune to these kinds of cultural messages, stories and expectations. In the words of one female participant in our research:

> I think that, women in the psych services, you become very conscious of your body image, because I've always had a figure, I was a size 12. By the time you've been on olanzapine for six months you are a size 18, so I think it's still something that society frowns upon and does make it quite hard for women. I don't like going swimming anymore because I feel like a large whale in my swimsuit.

As this excerpt suggests, anyone who believes her or his body does not conform to social expectations regarding slimness (or, for that matter, agility, skill, gender) may quite reasonably come to *feel* inadequate when entering a sport or physical activity space. Overcoming this feeling in order to initiate physical activity or sport participation can in itself be like climbing a mountain. While these kinds of experience can potentially affect *anybody*, it seems that women are particularly likely to be discouraged from participation as a result and, therefore, social expectations regarding body weight are a key factor in the lower sport and physical activity participation rates among women.

The knowledge that children build up in childhood, and the prejudices they adopt and sustain, are not restricted to simply fat and thin bodies. Children also learn that bodies are gendered and if they do not want to be considered 'deviant' then the games they play, the clothes they wear and the activities and sports they become involved with must align with what is culturally acceptable (Davies, 2001). Within Western society, girls who play 'boy's games' are frequently labelled 'tomboys' – not girls who like climbing trees, being active or competitive (Nelson, 1994). Until relatively recent times, girls and women were often *discouraged* from vigorous physical activity which builds muscle. Among women who have highly muscular physiques – for example female body builders – it is still not unusual for their gender and sexuality to be questioned because they transgress cultural expectations of femininity (Shilling & Bunsell, 2009).

For decades women have also been advised against vigorous activity on the basis that it damages the reproductive system and – even though recent research challenges this view – it is difficult to change beliefs that are embedded from childhood. Traditionally, these beliefs follow the plot of stories that portray girls as 'pretty princesses', feminine bodies as soft and smooth, and women as 'emotional' and in need of protection. In a similar vein, males who do not conform to symbolic markers of masculinity (e.g. a muscular, strong, dominating body) risk having their sexuality questioned (Madill & Hopper, 2007). Boys are encouraged to be 'courageous' and 'strong' and if they fail to exhibit these qualities attempts will be made by others to 'toughen them up' physically and emotionally (Dowling Naess, 2001).

These issues are important for practitioners to understand because gyms and sport centres are not neutral spaces. Particular messages about the body and health, about what it is to be male or female, are communicated via the stories and actions of people who work in and frequent these environments and by the narratives that underlie promotional literature. Although no formal, stated or enforced rules govern how an individual must present their body, there are serious consequences for those who transgress accepted norms and strong incentives to conform (Rudacille, 2006).

While in recent years greater investments have been made to increase participation in physical activity, the kinds of issues we have outlined above (which most certainly influence participation rates) are likely to increase an inactive person's anxiety about entering exercise spaces. These anxieties will not diminish simply because more money is being invested. If we are not to perpetuate damaging stereotypes and exclusion – devaluing those who do not conform to the ideal body – then considering *our* part in this culture is a priority. These points, we hope, serve as a reminder to all of us who work in mental health contexts that *everybody* who enters a physical activity space is likely to be influenced by cultural expectations concerning the body types that are promoted and valued, and the kinds of activities that are associated with achieving these aims.

The sporting landscape

Sport defines us as a nation. It teaches us about life. We learn self-discipline and teamwork from it. We learn how to win with grace and lose with dignity. It gets us fit. It keeps us healthy. It forms a central part of the cultural and recreational parts of our lives. (Department for Culture, Media and Sport, 2002)

The above statement is an illustration of the positive way sport is commonly promoted in contemporary Western cultures. From the governing bodies of sport to sport strategy documents, we learn that not only is sport fulfilling, healthy, lucrative and fun, but that it 'builds character', contributes to an individual's sense of identity and competence (Apitzsch, 1998), is empowering (Blinde *et al.*, 1994; Cantor & Bernay, 1992) and is a source of enjoyment (Bryson, 1987). It has been argued that not only does sport success build social esteem and self-esteem, it can also make entire nations 'feel good' and increase productivity. More recently, sport has also been promoted as a way to reduce crime and antisocial behaviour, to reduce social exclusion and to challenge racism (see Department for Culture, Media and Sport, 2002).

Although we agree that there are many potential benefits from becoming involved in sport – socially, physically and mentally – it is important to remember that sport culture is not without problems. Sport has a history of being elitist and many individuals have experienced exclusion from activities they would have liked to try. Sport also has a history of being sexist – both through banning women from playing certain sports and through condoning behaviours that are demeaning to women. Sport has also been a vehicle for sustaining hegemonic masculinity through endorsing aggressive behaviour and talk. An overly positive conception of sport among coaches, sport psychologists and enthusiasts has led some scholars to suggest that many practitioners have a 'default setting' which *blinds* them to these kinds of problems (Van Raalte & Anderson, 2007).

While many schools like to publicise their sport achievements, school sport also has a tainted history, being an activity many children dread. Adults with negative sport experiences in their childhood may never regain an interest or enthusiasm in any form of physical activity. Despite recent initiatives to make school sport appealing to *all* children, a report published by UK Sport observes that one in five girls say they take part in PE only because they have to, around 15% of girls do not enjoy PE and 30% of girls did not expect to be physically active when they leave school (UK Sport, 2006).

In describing the social cachet of the healthy body, we suggested that particular types of bodies are more highly valued than others in contemporary Western societies. Madill and Hopper (2007) note that the most highly valued *stories* in our culture are those where the primary character is powerful, strong and dominates others. They suggest that those who are involved in sport:

> draw on and are highly influenced by the role of the male professional athlete. Discourse surrounding professional athletes emphasises a hegemonic masculinity that promotes strength, power and war metaphors, and de-emphasises healthy lifestyle choices, such as exercise and food choices, sensitivity to others and appropriate social interaction in society. (p. 45)

While many people believe elite athletes make good role models, participation in elite and professional sport has also been associated with pathological development and a range of emotional and psychological problems which include alcohol and substance abuse, acute depression, eating disorders, identity confusion, suicidal ideation and de-creased self-confidence (see Ogilvie & Howe, 1982; Svoboda & Vanek, 1982; Blinde & Stratta, 1992; Sinclair & Orlick, 1993; Ogilvie, 1997; Sparkes, 1998; Sparkes & Douglas, 2007; Carless & Douglas, 2009a; Douglas & Carless, 2009a, 2009b).

In recent years, we detect a change of philosophy in sport, away from valuing taking part or simply 'playing the game', towards a stronger focus on *winning* and *winners*.

In the policy document *Playing to Win: A New Era for Sport* (Department for Culture, Media and Sport, 2008), the Secretary of State for Culture, Media and Sport writes:

> When you play sport, you play to win. That is my philosophy. It is also at the heart of this plan that, over time, seeks to change the culture of sport in England. It is a plan to get more people taking up sport simply for the love of sport; to expand the pool of talented English sportsmen and women; and to break records, win medals and win tournaments for this country.

This focus is not restricted to the UK, as indicated by the remarks of the Director of the Australian Institute of Sport (AIS) during a television interview in 2006:

> The main drive of the AIS is we are here to win. Getting a personal best and trying your hardest is fantastic and you would never knock an athlete for doing that, but you are here to win. Getting on the Olympic team is fantastic and getting a green and gold tracksuit is fantastic, but you're here to win. No athlete comes in here without fully understanding and being absolutely committed to winning, winning and winning. That's what it's all about.

While these philosophies may to some degree be expected in professional sport, they are not restricted to professional sport, as in children's sport and school sport too, performance outcomes (i.e. winning) increasingly seem to be the most highly prized outcome (see Ingham *et al.*, 2002).

In relation to this point, A Systematic Review of the Evidence Base for Developing a Physical Activity and Health Legacy from the London 2012 Olympic and Paralympic Games (Department of Health, 2009) unequivocally concludes that the 2012 Games (or any other major sports event) is not a 'magic bullet' which will increase participation in physical activity and sport, or encourage positive health behaviours. The report highlights that competitive sport at the elite level is not a particularly helpful model at the population level – high-level sport events are unlikely to turn inactive people into active people and are therefore unlikely to result in population health or lifestyle benefits. Any increases in sport and physical activity participation after major sport events, the report suggests, is likely to be limited to those who are already sport enthusiasts. On the one hand therefore we are bombarded by messages suggesting that sport/physical activity is a 'magic bullet' to increase participation (see, for example, Department for Culture, Media and Sport, 2008), while the unequivocal conclusions of some of the most educated and informed scholars in the field suggest it quite simply is not. Instead, as Patriksson (1995) reminds us, 'Sport, like most activities, is not a priori good or bad, but has the potential of producing both positive and negative outcomes' (Department for Culture, Media and Sport, 2002). With this point in mind, a key question we need to ask is: How might sport and physical activity provision be geared towards positive (rather than negative) outcomes?

Narrative types in sport and physical activity

One answer to the preceding question – which has become clear to us through our research with elite sportspeople (e.g. Douglas & Carless, 2006, 2009a; Carless &

Douglas, 2009a, 2009b) – is to consider the narratives (i.e. types of story) that circulate within sport and physical activity environments. As we discussed in chapter 2, stories play an important role in shaping people's experience. By attending to the stories that we ourselves tell – and the ways we respond to others' stories – we have an opportunity to exert a positive influence on the sport and physical activity experiences of those with whom we work.

The performance narrative

Within sport settings, we have proposed that a particular narrative type is dominant: the *performance* narrative (see Douglas & Carless, 2006). It is a story where performance outcomes are central and, in its ideal form, is a type of 'hero narrative' where the hero overcomes obstacles to reach their goal, which usually involves winning through competition. Performance stories often include talk of skills, talent, charting progress, medals, cups, trophies and other performance outcomes. The following extract, taken from an interview with a professional golfer, provides the flavour of a typical performance narrative:

> I just love sport, any sport. You introduce me to any sport and I'll have a go. I just like competition – I suppose to see how good you can actually be, so you can stretch yourself. I need to stretch myself to see how capable I am. I need competition – that's what it is, that's what you chose to go into. At the end of the day there is a trophy and there is a cheque and another notch in how many wins you've had. A lot of it is about winning. (Douglas & Carless, 2006, p. 19)

This extract shows how – while competition is important – it is the *outcome* of competition which is critical: for those who tell performance tales, positive feelings come through *winning*.

This in itself is not necessarily a problem, provided positive feelings can also be experienced through other avenues. Most of us enjoy winning from time to time and taking a trophy or medal home is a symbolic acknowledgement of an achievement. The drive to win can be problematic though when it becomes the *only* story that an individual can create and develop. This is the case in the performance narrative where being 'successful' is cast as requiring an overriding focus on one's sport. For example:

> I say that the person and the job and the person and the golf go together. I couldn't be successful without it being the most important thing in my life. My golf is more important than anything. If I was in a relationship I would have to say to whoever that was, this is huge – it is not a job. It's much more than that. It is not just a career. I think that all of us, it becomes our whole life. Because I don't think that you can possibly be successful without it being the most important thing. (Douglas & Carless, 2006, p. 20)

The single-minded nature of this excerpt reveals an overriding focus on sport performance to the exclusion of all other areas of life and self. This, for us, is dangerous because identity and self-worth becomes dependent on performance outcomes. One athlete described the personal effects of being knocked out (missing the 'cut') of a golf tournament:

> When I missed those cuts I felt dreadful about myself. I was letting everybody down and myself. I had no self-esteem, everything just went, totally. I was distraught. What do you do? You know, you feel lower and lower about yourself. It was just a nightmare. Huge. I think I just lost all my confidence in one round of golf. (Douglas & Carless, 2006, p. 20)

As this excerpt suggests, there is a very real risk for those who tell performance stories that when performance fails (e.g. because a person stops winning, is injured or retires from sport), so does the self. Should poor performances continue, shame, self-doubt, depression and identity collapse are potential outcomes (see Sparkes, 1998; Carless & Douglas 2009a; Douglas & Carless, 2009a).

In exercise settings, the performance narrative is likely to take a slightly different form where the teller's focus is on reaching their target weight or finishing their exercise plan and moving to the next level. As such, it is a monadic story where the teller's focus is on the self. By this we mean that their stories are of *my* weight, *my* blood pressure, *my* bone mineral density, *my* fat to weight ratio, *my* exercise plan. Should these outcomes come to dominate a person's life then the kinds of dangers we have described in a sport setting become a potential threat.

Performance stories do have a role to play in helping some individuals give voice to their experience. For some people who want to lose weight, increase their strength or coordination or play in competitions, the performance narrative provides a template to help them narrate their experience. There is a danger though that, by being accepted and promoted as the *only* way to be involved in sport or exercise, the performance narrative silences alternatives. That is, other philosophies or different ways to approach sport or physical activity risk being misunderstood, trivialised, villainised or denied. For example, stories along the lines of 'I just play for fun' or 'I just like the drink with my mates in the bar afterwards' come to be viewed (from the perspective of the performance narrative) as incompatible with 'success' and therefore disparaged or discouraged.

Alternative narrative types

It is, of course, possible to engage in physical activity or sport at *any* level without aligning with the performance narrative. We have identified two alternative narrative types among elite sportspeople: the *discovery* and the *relational* narrative (Douglas & Carless, 2006).

In the discovery narrative the storyteller describes discovering and exploring a life full of people, places and experiences using sport as a conduit to achieve these aims. Discovery stories are characterised by talk about learning new skills and enjoying experiences which are not related to performance outcomes, such as travel, meeting new people or going to new places. In this tale, sport is considered one part of a full, rich and multidimensional life. Tellers of discovery tales might recount achieving success without prioritising sport over other areas of life and typically describe the maintenance and development of other roles, identities and interests as complementary to (rather than impeding) their involvement in sport. In a discovery story, self-worth is not dependent on sport achievement, but supported by a broad range of life roles and activities.

In the relational narrative the central focus is on interdependent connection/s between two or more people in which sport performance is essentially a by-product. Relational stories typically tell of doing sport or activity with parents, siblings, a partner, friends, and so on. Tellers of these stories adopt an empathic awareness of other people's needs, of engaging in the activity *with* a significant other or *for* another person. These stories value relationship/s with others over and above performance outcomes, so being with others is storied as more important than achievement, success, trophies or glory. Altruistic rather than ego motivation dominates this type of story and the storyteller is likely to place the perceived needs of others above the needs of the self.

The presence of these alternatives is, we think, important. The performance narrative dominates sport and exercise culture: it is promoted and publicised in the sport press, in television coverage of sport events, through interviews with many sporting celebrities. It is – in many quarters – assumed to be *the only way* through which it is possible to be 'successful' in sport. On this basis, it needs no further support or promotion by sport coaches, exercise leaders, personal trainers or health professionals. It is *alternative* types of story – such as discovery and relational narratives – that need to be legitimised, supported, nurtured and encouraged. It is these story types, our research suggests, that hold the key to beneficial and healthful sport and physical activity.

By becoming aware of alternatives to the performance narrative practitioners have the chance to be open to, and accepting of, diversity among the individuals with whom they work. As Frank (1995) suggests, becoming familiar with alternative narratives help us to more effectively 'hear', understand and respond to personal stories which do not 'fit' with the story we were expecting. If we are aware of alternative narratives, we are less likely to subconsciously 'miss', 'silence' or 'suppress' an individual's story which contravenes the script of the performance narrative. This is a useful process because: (i) personal stories help us get to know and understand the teller because a person's stories reveal their history, preferences, needs, identity and aspirations; and (ii) being familiar with the plots of different narrative types enables us to understand and prepare for the possible consequences of individuals' personal stories.

An example might clarify these points. Health and fitness practitioners who align with a performance narrative are likely to evaluate the 'success' of a client solely on the basis of performance outcomes: by establishing if they adhered to the exercise plan or remain on track to reach their goal weight. By doing so, a host of other possible reasons for exercise (such as exploration, development, relationships) are missed. There is a risk that practitioners who align with the performance narrative will thereby show a lack of understanding for individuals who are more inclined towards a discovery or relational orientation. At times, this lack of interest or understanding may even be enacted as a disparaging attitude towards those who are disinterested in – or unable to achieve – particular performance outcomes.

To compensate for a cultural bias towards performance-oriented stories, we suggest that practitioners focus their efforts on promoting and legitimising discovery and re-lational stories while downplaying performance stories. Several strategies are likely to prove useful in this regard:

- Try to reflect on your own talk, conversation and verbal interaction: what kind of narrative underlies your stories? Do you espouse performance values (i.e.

winning, competition, dedication, single-mindedness)? Do you support and encourage discovery narratives through sharing stories of exploration, learning, personal development, growth? Do you facilitate relational narratives through sharing stories of social connectedness, friendship, cooperation?

■   Consider your own position on the diverse reasons people may have for becoming involved in sport or physical activity. Does your provision cater for non-performance goals? Is the way you publicise or advertise sessions likely to appeal to individuals who may have had bad experiences of competitive sport (perhaps at school) but would like to re-engage in order to meet new people or learn new skills?

■   The physical environment, organisation and delivery of sessions are all likely to influence the stories that individuals feel able to create and share. To this end, can competition (especially with others) be minimised or downplayed in favour of new learning and experiences (e.g. through a guided discovery approach to coaching) or relationship building (e.g. through cooperative team activities)?

Key points

■   Our aim with this chapter has not been to extol the virtues of physical activity and sport, nor simply define the problems. Rather, we have tried to reveal how sport and physical activity can have negative as well as positive outcomes which are strongly influenced by socio-cultural factors, expectations and norms. From this perspective, the stories *we* tell (as coaches, exercise leaders, and so on) about sport and physical activity make a difference to the kinds of experience individuals are likely to have.

■   We have proposed that a particular narrative type – a performance narrative (which focuses on competition and winning) – dominates sport and physical activity culture. This narrative provides a particular script for sport and activity experience which is only workable when an individual is winning (in sport) or sticking to training (at the gym). At other times, this type of story can have damaging effects on individual well-being and self-worth. We suggest that, given the cultural dominance of this story type, it needs no further promotion through sport/exercise provision in mental health.

■   We identified two alternative narrative types – discovery and relational narratives – which provide different scripts by which individuals might experience sport and activity. These alternative stories provide an opportunity for others to hear and create a story which may better fit their own experience and aspirations. The values and behaviours inherent in the discovery and relational stories, we suggest, are more likely to lead to positive long-term psychological outcomes and personal development. These narrative types might therefore be beneficially encouraged and supported in sport and physical activity contexts related to mental health.

■   It is a concern that there seems to be a common belief among practitioners in sport and exercise that there is only *one* type of social experience and that all athletes, exercisers, body-builders, runners, walkers, cyclists and so on hold the same values, ideals and goals. This is not the case as great diversity exists in terms of what individuals seek through sport or activity involvement. There is therefore a need for practitioners to acknowledge difference without devaluing alternative motives and aims. It is necessary that as sport and exercise practitioners we consider our own biases and possible blindness in order to recognise how we may extend provision to better meet the needs of diverse persons with differing needs and aspirations.

Women in sport and physical activity

Many of us experience situations where we *can't see the wood for the trees*, when we recognise something is wrong, but fail to change in response. In the seventeenth century, Galileo faced an inquisition for challenging the view that the earth was flat and located at the centre of the universe. At this point in history, 'male-centred' views about the world – and women's place in it – were also widely accepted and yet to be challenged. What was assumed then about women would probably now sound as absurd as the belief that the earth is flat. Yet, because what was 'known' about women and about science originated from powerful, educated men, it came to be accepted as 'the truth'. It has taken decades and huge investments for humankind to better understand the cosmos – and it has taken decades and the huge personal sacrifice of many women to begin to show that scientists have too often done a disservice to women by perpetuating myths about the female body and its potential.

In this chapter, we reconsider the prevailing approach towards the provision and promotion of sport and exercise which we suggest tends to devalue or ignore some women's motives and ways of being. Sport (and, arguably, exercise too) has historically been an area where the masculine values of power, domination, individuation and competition are seen as central and intrinsic to sport itself. While these values are acceptable to many sport enthusiasts, they are not necessarily acceptable to many women. When these values are wholeheartedly encouraged among those who do not currently engage in sport and physical activity, it should not be surprising that sport and physical activity promotion fails. In this chapter we explore an alternative orientation which, to some, might seem as radical as Galileo's claim that the earth is a sphere. By doing so, we offer one answer to the question of why sport and physical activity participation rates among women remain lower than among men, and suggest some ways through which better sport and physical activity provision might be made for women in mental health contexts.

The state of play

Over the past decade we have delivered a number of continuing professional development (CPD) workshops and seminars for sport coaches. Although we have worked with practitioners across different sport and physical activity settings, our CPD work began among professional golf coaches. Notable in the workshops for the Professional Golfers Association (PGA) – by their *absence* – were female golf coaches. From time to time, one or two female coaches attended a course but, by and large over an eight-year period, the vast majority of delegates were male. Given that the hierarchy of most sport organisations in the UK is male and that the majority of coaches are also male (UK Sport, 2006), our experiences of all-male groups was no big surprise.

One reason for the low percentage of females taking coaching and leadership roles in sport is that female participation in sport has also historically been low (Department for Culture Media and Sport, 2002; UK Sport, 2006). This is a factor which we feel has also impinged on our research in mental health. Relatively few women took part in regular sport or exercise sessions at the day centre where we carried out our research – this was typified in a golf project we ran (see Carless & Douglas, 2004 and chapter 11) where all participants were male.

The coaches who attended the seminars we conducted for the PGA were not unaware that female participation rates are low in golf (85% of club members are male). While a few professionals appeared disinterested in improving the situation, many demonstrated a commitment to encourage more women and girls into golf and many appeared to be frustrated that many girls dropped out after appearing to enjoy playing and improving their games. During the seminars, after discussing feminist research which explored women's motivation and participation in sport, we would ask coaches to reflect on their own experience. Many concluded that their male and female pupils exhibited some notable differences that went beyond anatomy and biology. For example, some shared stories about female students who did not want to take lessons alone but were at ease taking group lessons. Coaches did not generally report such a strong desire to be with friends among male students. Some noted that whereas many girls appeared content 'sitting and chatting', boys often wouldn't sit still, and would be hitting shots long before they were instructed to do so. Some coaches recounted stories of female pupils being disappointed if they progressed to a higher skilled group for coaching when it meant they were to be separated from their friends. In contrast boys often appeared to relish progression. Although many coaches noticed these and other differences, this awareness had brought few adjustments to their coaching practice.

Feminist researchers have shown that many mainstream sports have been organised and run along a model that fits masculine interests. As governments have begun to consider the health and social costs of excluding women, and research has made more obvious the way women and girls have been discouraged from engagement, substantial investments have been targeted in the UK at major sports with the aim of changing the situation and increasing the number of women and girls who participate. This has led to changes to the law and at times the threat of withdrawal of funding, in attempts to encourage sport hierarchies to improve provision for women. Despite the investments, however, research carried out by the Youth Sport Trust (Nike/Youth Sport Trust, 2006) shows that one in five children believe it is not important for girls to be good at sport, nor is 'being sporty' an image that is 'cool' for girls. Forty percent of girls continue to feel self-conscious when participating in sport and physical activity and a good number find sport boring.

These findings mirror research among older women where ageing does not appear to diminish negative feelings about the body in physical activity contexts nor ameliorate a perception that gyms and exercise classes are boring (Women's Sport Foundation, 2005). It appears that, irrespective of changes to the law, progressive inclusive strategies and huge investments, fundamental barriers to participation remain for some women. It seems that some assumptions about what sport is or what it is believed to be, something about the *way* sport and physical activities are run – and the way they are promoted – is unappealing to these individuals. On this basis, merely making existing provision available to women, or simply starting a women's football group, or women's rugby group, is not enough: in order to reach those who are currently not physically active, a different approach is needed. To explore what form this approach might take, we turn now to the stories women tell of their sport and physical activity experiences.

Women's stories of physical activity and sport

We create an identity (a sense of who we are as a person) through the process of creating and sharing stories of our life. Through telling stories about the things we do, a particular identity begins to take shape: an individual who 'likes' one thing, but knows that another thing 'is not me'. In striving to achieve a *coherent* identity, we tend to link our actions over time in ways that fit with a bigger life story. By doing so, we bring a sense of continuity to our lives across time, and reveal how the identity we have created informs our subsequent actions and behaviours. Knowing who we are provides the basis of knowing how to act in the future and helps us decide the types of actions we wish to invest ourselves in.

These narrative processes help us understand women's experiences of sport and physical activity. If we want to support a woman to participate, then as practitioners we need to offer the opportunity for actions which align with her identity – rather than threaten or compromise her identity. For example, if a young woman holds the belief that to 'be a woman' is to be slim and unmuscular, she is unlikely to attend a weight-lifting class. If however, the same woman gains an understanding that to 'be female' is to be strong, decisive and athletic, then she is more likely to engage in weight training.

When we asked women in professional sport to describe their reasons for playing sport, three different types of narrative were evident: performance, discovery and relational narratives (see Douglas & Carless, 2006 and chapter 7). Looking across the landscape of human experience, each of these narrative types might be valued in some contexts, but unexpected in others. In sport, it is the performance narrative that dominates to the extent that this story is very often *expected*. In our research among older women (Douglas & Carless, 2005), however, the dominant narrative was a relational narrative. In many of these women's stories, physical activity was not described in terms of *performance outcomes*, but rather in terms of *relationships*.

A typical example was provided by Sophia, a 70-year-old woman who talked about – as a child – playing sport *with* her brother and friends, doing chores in the house *for* her mother, working on a farm *for* her family (because they had little money) when she should have been going to school. Sophia's *with* and *for* stories were rooted in her childhood yet they continued to shape her actions in the present day. They illustrate that for Sophia, like many women, their actions – be it playing sport or physical labour – took place because of relationships and attachments, because of care for and connection to other people. Absent from these stories was talk about getting fitter, being competitive, or winning medals. Although these outcomes might have occurred, they were not the main plot of the story, which focused instead on *connection* to others. This focus is central to the relational narrative and contrasts dramatically to the values of the performance narrative with its emphasis on the self.

Relational stories were told time and time again by the older women in our research and helped us understand their participation in physical activity. When activity was perceived to lead only or primarily to performance outcomes (e.g. improved fitness through solitary exercise in the gym), it was unappealing and participation would not be maintained. If, however, an activity facilitated or supported valued relationships, then participation was more likely. As a result, even when an activity wasn't particularly appealing, an individual could be 'roped in' by a family member or friend. We learnt how if an activity lost its appeal, a woman might continue because she attended the activity with a friend. Going back to our example of Sophia, she described in great detail her love of dancing – the skills and joy this activity brought her, the fun she had with a group of friends each week. But she also described days in the winter when it was cold, wet and she didn't want to go. At these times she described very clearly that what motivated her was 'knowing her friend would want to go', and that if she didn't go then her friend wouldn't be able to go.

In these instances, women revealed a strong orientation towards the well-being, needs and care of another person. Such an orientation – playing sport for another person or going to a dancing class for another person – might appear quite foreign to those individuals who participate in physical activity on the basis of personal performance outcomes. Because a relational orientation is not well understood it is not catered for in most sport and exercise contexts; relational narratives are often inadvertently devalued and trivialised in the promotion of sport and physical activity. Yet these relational attachments, we suggest, are at the core of many women's motivation. Outside of sport and physical activity contexts, for example, in motherhood and nursing, it is expected for women to tell stories which focus on the well-being of others, yet few people in sport and physical activity contexts make the connection that the person is unlikely to change simply because they are faced with a different activity.

Among the older women in our research, age had not rewritten the values and identities which directed their actions across the landscape of their lives. It is therefore important to recognise that when relationally motivated individuals are asked to put their own needs before the needs of significant others, they are not simply being asked to adopt a 'change of behaviour', but rather, they are being asked to change a valued dimension of the *self* and, quite possibly, *lose* a valuable component of their *identity*.

We are not so much suggesting that one type of narrative is *better* but, rather, that when one type of narrative silences alternative stories it can be damaging in terms of participation. Physical activity and sport programmes which are talked about, promoted and organised around what they can do for the *self* are unlikely to appeal to those who are oriented to the needs of the *other*. On this basis, it is important that practitioners in sport and exercise recognise, value and provide for individuals who are more inclined towards the relational ways of being. We suspect that many women who are resistant to sport and physical activity fall into this category.

Practitioner blindness

A current 'problem' within sport is that the performance narrative heavily influences promotion, education, practice and provision of physical activity and sport to the extent that the assumptions some practitioners hold blind them to alternatives. When we are able to identify different narrative types, it is possible to appreciate how people who may appear similar have very different orientations in life. When asked to illustrate this point we usually use the analogy of a map. Looking at a map of the UK, for example, there is a choice of possible routes to drive from Bristol to Glasgow. If the objective of the journey was to get to Glasgow *quickly*, the 'best' route would be up the motorway. The motorway system, however, is but one possible route. If another person's objective was to get to Glasgow *enjoyably*, he or she may decide to go via the Welsh countryside or the Lake District. In doing so they would experience breathtaking scenery, ancient castles and quite possibly hear a different language being spoken when they stopped for petrol. If enjoyment, personal development and rewarding experiences were the priority, the 'best' route would be the longer slower route. In a similar way, when we become more aware of alternative narrative types it can help us better understand and provide for individuals whose motives, interests and values may differ from our own.

Carole Gilligan (1993) has drawn attention to the ways that women's voices and stories have been systematically silenced by traditional psychological approaches to identity and development. For Gilligan, 'The failure to hear the differences in their voices stems in part from the assumption that there is a single mode of social experience and interpretation' (p. 173). Likewise, Bakan (1966) and McAdams (2001) have described different ways of 'being' in the world. One way of being (which aligns with the performance narrative) is characterised by a tendency to separate self from others, to gain agency and status and to dominate others. Another (which aligns with a relational narrative type) is characterised by an orientation towards unity, communion, friendship and caring for others. Gergen (1999) suggests theories which consider people to possess a unified ego – to all 'be' a certain way – are dangerous because they blind those who hold such a view to alternative ways of being. If we said that the *only* permitted way to drive to Glasgow is via the motorway, some people would not bother making the trip. Yet, this is what happens all too frequently in sport and physical activity settings as we offer what – to some people – appears to be a 'quick trip to boredom'.

This point has been illustrated to us in CPD seminars when we have presented our research to professional golf coaches (Douglas & Carless, 2008a). The delegates (experienced, qualified professional coaches at level 3 or above) were accepting of the story plot which they *expected* to hear: the performance narrative. In contrast, when presented with alternative narrative types (the discovery and relational narrative), they often responded with disbelief. Many believed it to be *impossible* to get to the top in sport without solely focusing on winning. This is because the route that is mapped out for this type of journey (to get to the top in sport) assumes all athletes have a similar orientation in life. Many coaches were shocked by a top pro saying 'I did it for dad.' Many seemed openly dumbfounded that a tournament winner could say that winning the trophy was less important than doing something which made someone else happy. Most of these coaches had been schooled to think that in sport you have to do it for yourself and that not to be self-focused in this regard would negatively influence performance. Likewise, when we have presented these different story plots to sport and health science students there is a general acceptance of the performance narrative (as 'the way it is') and surprise that alternatives exist.

In 2008, Kitrina was commissioned to evaluate a manual for cardiac rehabilitation patients. The manual, which included a six-week rehabilitation course, provided patients with information about the causes of a heart attack, the difficulties they may subsequently experience, and an exercise plan to follow at home. The steering group were interested to explore how effective the manual was for increasing home-based physical activity among cardiac patients. One theme which Kitrina noted in every interview and focus group conducted with cardiac nurses, community nurses and physiotherapists, was that practitioners did not understand why so many patients did not lose weight or take more exercise. The story plot these practitioners seemed to expect was one where following a heart attack patients would follow exercise recommendations *in an effort to improve their own fitness/health*. This is the plot of a performance narrative: it focuses solely or primarily on *me* achieving a particular performance outcome (i.e. fitness) in the context of *my own life*. Because they were not aware of other possible stories, practitioners tended to 'judge' those who did not adhere to the exercise programme as 'a failure' or even 'deviant'. As a result, practitioners failed to consider other reasons why patients did not engage with the exercise regime.

Through considering alternative narrative types – in this case a relational narrative – it is possible to identify a story plot through which the teller remains inactive yet is not a 'failure' or 'deviant'. Whereas the performance narrative aligns with Western culture's interest in the *self*, the relational narrative plot centres on relational dimensions of life: the *other*. In this regard attachment and affiliation are valued as highly – or more highly – than self-enhancement (see Miller, 1976; Gilligan, 1993; Josselson, 1996). In the case of the heart manual, a large number of the individuals who experienced a heart attack were themselves carers and, despite becoming unwell, continued to care for a family member. People who create a sense of self and identity which is oriented towards the needs of another are used to putting another's needs above their own. From a relational perspective – where the major concern is not the self but the other – this behaviour is entirely understandable and authentic, especially if the new exercise regime threatens time that is normally spent with or caring for a significant other.

Improving provision for women in mental health contexts

We do not wish to suggest that *all* women's stories will conform to the relational narrative. Neither do we wish to suggest that *no* men will tell relational stories. Instead, we suggest that among those women who *do not currently take part* in sport or physical activity, a relational orientation is likely to be common. For these individuals, the dominant performance stories have limited appeal. Viewed from this perspective, if we, as practitioners, hope to encourage individuals who align with a relational narrative to participate in physical activity or sport some new approaches are needed. These might include:

- *Talking about sport/physical activity in relational way.* Coaches and leaders often ask performance-focused questions (e.g. Did you win? What time did you do?) which lead people towards a performance focus. This is likely to be unappealing to some women. By asking instead relational questions (e.g. Who did you meet at the session? Did you have any good conversations? Did you help anyone?), a relational orientation is suggested which is likely to be more appealing to some women.
- *Include significant others where possible.* Physical activity and sport initiatives which are geared to include existing family, friends and significant others are more likely to interest currently inactive women with a relational orientation. Others might be included in the activity itself, in a social component accompanying the activity or through talking about and sharing stories of activity experiences.
- *Tailor the activity towards relational processes and outcomes.* Consider structuring the activity around opportunities for social interaction and connection. Possible strategies include: incorporating social time before/during/after the session perhaps through refreshment breaks; emphasising cooperative (rather than competitive) activities which bring people together and encourage people to work together; including opportunities for peer coaching and support where group members are encouraged to interact in order to help each other progress. Having an orientation to others needs means that individuals who are relationally focused may respond to helping coach or lead the session as this may provide an opportunity to *give* to others.
- *Choose 'relationship-friendly' activities.* Dance activities (for example) require individuals to move *together* as a group. Unlike most sports, which require an individual to be *against* others, dance complements the types of identity and self that many women have created through their lives because it allows an individual to be *with* and *for* others. Many women describe the importance of dancing in their lives, irrespective of whether they have a sport background or not. Dance has only recently been included on Sport England's radar as an activity with mass appeal and that is also of particular interest to females. In any context, therefore, where physical activity sessions are to be staged, not to include some types of dance-based activity shows a lack of awareness of women's interests.
- *Evaluate the activity in terms of relational processes and outcomes as opposed to performance processes and outcomes.* Rather than setting outcome goals related to performance (e.g. weight loss, fitness improvement, tournament position, distance walked), is it possible to create relational goals? Possible ideas include the quality and quantity of social events, interactions with others, new partners/teams played with or against.
- *It's not only about the game or match.* For some people, it is not important to play a game or a match, 'just' playing is enough. Too frequently, our talk about these individuals ('they're *only* knocking up') suggests that playing is in some way inferior to or less important than competition. As practitioners we need to remember that

some people are enriched by throwing a frisbee, hitting a shuttle back and forth, running about, knocking a ball against a wall, and so on. It is important that these ways of playing are not devalued and that these individuals are not pushed to the sidelines or their play confined to the fringes of competition.

Key points

- We have suggested that some women (and some men too) are oriented towards a *relational* way of being which is not well catered for within existing sport and exercise provision which tends to assume a *performance* orientation. To provide sport and physical activity opportunities which will appeal to these individuals, practitioners need to rethink provision away from performance outcomes and towards the development and maintenance of relationships.
- When sport or physical activity is promoted on the basis of what it contributes to a woman's health, it will only be appealing to those who attach primary importance to their own health. Among the women in our research, many prioritised relationships with their partner, children, grandchildren, siblings, parents or close friends ahead of their own health. For these women, identity and self is created and sustained only within webs of connection. Activity programmes which threaten or fail to cater for these connections and relationships are unlikely to be experienced as beneficial.
- For relationally oriented individuals, relationships and webs of connection need to be incorporated into sport and physical activity settings. For some, the relationship with the exercise leader and/or other group members might be the most important part of the sport session, not the activity itself. The session leader or coach is therefore a facilitator of *with* and *for* opportunities, not just the expert in physical and technical requirements of the activity. In this regard, a key aim for coaches is creating time to talk, time to share a coffee or cold drink, time to share a laugh, and time to share experiences that cannot be shared outside the mental health setting. These goals need not prevent sport-specific skills being learned or achievement and progression being supported.
- While this chapter has been devoted to *women's* involvement in physical activity and sport, we recognise that some men too may be relationally oriented. On this basis, we advocate moving away from gender distinctions and see all activities as potentially appropriate for either gender. We would make no distinctions about the applicability of dance for men or weight-lifting for women. Our point is that it is the *way* in which the activity is organised and the values which underpin provision (i.e. performance or relational) that will affect the degree to which it appeals to those who are currently not taking part in sport or physical activity.

Social support for participation 9

Successful physical activity or sport programmes in mental health settings are dependent on a number of ingredients in order to be effective. One of these ingredients is social support, widely recognised as an important factor in recovery (e.g. Corrigan & Phelan, 2004; Davidson *et al.*, 2005) and, as Anthony (1993) has observed, 'most first-person accounts of recovery from catastrophe (including mental illness) recount the critical nature of social support' (p. 22). It is also an important factor in successful exercise initiation and maintenance among the general population as well as people referred to exercise programmes on the basis of physical health concerns (Crone *et al.*, 2005). Among people with serious mental illness, the provision of adequate social support has been documented as a fundamental requirement for initiation and sustained participation, as 'the symptoms of mental illness combined with the side-effects of anti-psychotic medication make the initiation and maintenance of new activities such as exercise challenging for mental health service users and mental health professionals alike' (Carless, 2007, p. 18).

In recognition of these challenges, Richardson and colleagues (2005, p. 327) emphasise the important and diverse roles that exercise leaders need to take, saying 'Enthusiastic, knowledgeable, and supportive exercise leaders are as important as the actual exercise prescription itself.' In a similar vein, through their focus group research with outpatients in psychiatric rehabilitation, McDevitt and colleagues (2006) identify three ways in which support can help individuals overcome the barriers to regular physical activity:

(1) *Motivational leadership* – in the shape of the 'right kind' of leader who believes in them and that they could successfully engage in activity.
(2) *Relevant information* – which participants noted could 'give you the drive to do things' if they understood how following health recommendations could help them.

(3) *Group support, individual options* – through the provision of group activities which increase motivation and fun without sacrificing individual choice and flexibility.

In our view, various forms of social support are likely to be a prerequisite for successful physical activity and sport participation for the majority of people, whether or not they are experiencing mental health difficulties. Given its importance, in this chapter we explore the intricacies of social support provision in mental health contexts by focusing on a multidimensional model of social support developed by Rees and Hardy (2000). We have incorporated this model within our own research in mental health (see Carless & Douglas, 2008c) and address in turn each of the four forms of social support which comprise the model. Our purpose here is to consider practical strategies which are likely to be useful in physical activity, sport and mental health contexts.

Informational support

Informational support has been described as the task of 'providing the individual with advice or guidance concerning possible solutions to a problem' (Rees *et al.*, 2003, p. 137). Often informational support is the first form of support to be offered, generally on a one-to-one basis and typically before an individual actually becomes involved in the activity or sport. In this guise, social support is provided for potential exercisers through the provision of information about the benefits of the sport or activity which might be relevant to their personal needs or aspirations. The information offered is usually simple, practical and individual-specific, as one individual's description of how he began an exercise programme suggest: 'They [two physiotherapists] made a programme for me and I started ... I think they asked me what I wanted to do, then they just told me what was available and what I could fit in, like a school programme.' The following extract from one physiotherapist describes one strategy for providing initial informational support:

> What we do with everybody who comes is I just sort of go and have a chat with them and I've got a ... 'fit to begin' questionnaire and [I] go through that with each person and see if they want to join in any sports groups or use the exercise equipment here.

As this excerpt illustrates, the purpose of initial discussion was to present the activity as *possible*, *potentially beneficial* and *personally relevant* in some way. Through raising awareness of the potential benefits of the activity, informational support helps stimulate an individual's interest and motivation to get started with a particular exercise or activity.

Informational support is often also in evidence during activity sessions (in the form of teaching or coaching pointers), when a qualified coach or exercise practitioner is present. In our experience, this kind of support is often perceived to be valuable especially when it comes from someone who is themselves qualified and skilled, and can expand the knowledge and understanding of participants about the activity, as the following remarks from members of a golf group illustrate:

David: *What about the teaching ... has that been a good thing or would you rather you didn't get that?*

Yeah, it's been quite helpful. I wouldn't have figured out on my own about keeping your arm straight, and the way to hold the club. So I think it's helpful. Just want a few tips and then try them out.

Kitrina: Can you just tell me about the teaching, particularly, that you received?
Yeah. It was very good tuition actually 'cause it helped me improve my driving shots.

The provision of personally relevant and accessible informational support (through appropriate teaching or coaching input) seems to be important as it provides individuals with practical strategies which help develop their ability and skills and, subsequently, increase their confidence and enjoyment of the activity.

Significantly, we have also seen how informational support is often not only given *to* participants *by* a health professional or coach, but also *shared between* group members. In these scenarios a group member may provide information about a particular problem another person is experiencing or temporarily assume the role of teacher or coach by offering technical input.

This type of support is not restricted to information about fitness, health or sport. A care co-ordinator, for example, described how members of a football group provided 'informal' informational support to one individual concerning financial issues such as managing his credit card. This information is typically provided in an informal way that most of us experience during 'off-the-game' conversations in sport. Sport-specific informational support is not only provided by those who run and coach sessions; at times it is also provided *by* a participant *for* a mental health professional. One mental health professional described how William (a client) helped Julian (a mental health professional) with his golf: 'Last week he [William] played with Julian and was coaching him all the way round. So he was in his element 'cause ultimately that's what he wants to do. It worked out really well.'

We believe the importance of two-way sharing – giving and receiving – shouldn't be underestimated as it is significant in all of our lives. However, in taking such a stance there is a need for a slight change in perspective on the part of the group leader, exercise specialist or coach. Their role is also to recognise and value what others might bring to a session, as opposed to only considering that they are there to receive. In acknowledging that others in the group have the potential to give, their input can be beneficially nurtured and encouraged in sport or activity contexts.

Tangible support

Tangible support is described as 'concrete instrumental assistance, in which a person in a stressful situation is given the necessary resources (e.g., financial assistance, physical help with tasks) to cope with the stressful event' (Rees *et al.*, 2003, p. 137). In our experience, tangible support often has a simple but powerful effect on physical activity and sport participation. Its importance is most clearly evidenced in the form of financial assistance and the provision of basic needs such as transport which serve to minimise the barriers participants face in accessing sport and activity facilities. The importance of tangible support is illustrated, for example, in the following exchanges with two members of a golf group:

Kitrina: How do you think that we could develop the golf project? What would you like to see done?

Um (pause). I don't know really. Uh (pause). Cause it's the transport side really.

Kitrina: So for you, what are the difficulties that you face in playing? (pause) Transport's one of them?

Transport's one of them … getting out there. That's the main thing. And the fees is another one.

Kitrina: How much it costs?

How much it costs.

David: You don't want to join a golf club?

It's too expensive isn't it, yeah.

David: Do you think that's the main problem that you face?

Yeah, yeah.

These examples draw attention to the unavoidable impact of the *absence* or *lack* of tangible support: these participants communicated the view that exercise or sport would simply not happen without the provision of a basic level of tangible support. Most often, the tangible support required is assistance with transportation and a fairly modest level of funding to cover the direct costs of participation in the activity (e.g. entry to the exercise facility, hire of equipment).

In the case of one particular sport group, mental health professionals felt that the provision of free transport helped to increase participation. As one put it, 'It was made quite easy for them, you know, a minibus was provided and so they just had to kind of turn up.' According to another:

> The minibus was probably very important … 'cause our client group just won't, well they do, people do get to places on their own but they don't … certain people like Ronnie and William probably wouldn't have got there if they hadn't had a lift from their home to the centre.

In the case of the golf project therefore, the withdrawal of tangible support, through an absence of ongoing funding for this particular activity, was seen by staff and clients alike as the primary reason why golf participation would be threatened. As one staff member put it:

> Money is a major thing, they wouldn't go out and do it 'cause of money basically. Yeah, one comment was, can't remember who it was from, they wouldn't do this because it would cost too much and they wouldn't be able to afford it.

We suggest that financial support is likely to be essential in activities such as golf, where socioeconomic obstacles faced by many people with severe and enduring mental health problems make participation impossible.

Esteem support

Esteem support is described as 'the bolstering of a person's sense of competence or self-esteem by other people. Giving an individual positive feedback on his or her skills and abilities or expressing a belief that the person is capable of coping with a stressful event are examples of this type of support' (Rees *et al.*, 2003, p. 137). One participant's description of the support he received from staff during his initial exercise sessions provides a clear illustration of the importance and value of esteem support:

> If it wasn't for Sarah and Catherine I don't think I'd have got back into it. Well, I would have got back into it, but not so soon ... I think it was important for them to be there first of all. It gave me a bit of confidence. Because I was so unwell, I had no confidence, thinking I was gonna have a panic attack, stuff like that ... somebody there I could chat to and take my mind off it.

This excerpt provides an illustration of the importance and value of esteem support, and how a person who is perceived as a knowledgeable person (in this case a physiotherapist) can – just by being there – instil confidence and security for an activity which an individual is afraid may lead to an adverse consequence. Additionally by being, in this participant's words, 'somebody I could chat to' the physiotherapists had an opportunity to promote the individual's self-efficacy for the particular activity through a process of *verbal persuasion*. In this example, esteem support was provided through a process of verbal interaction which mitigated the individual's doubts and concerns regarding his ability to engage in the activity.

Another participant illustrates the powerful effects of this type of esteem support by describing how '[I was] a bit slow to start with. But Sarah said you'll improve as you go along ... it was true.' For many individuals, simple but positive comments from exercise leaders are valuable, particularly during the early stages of involvement, because they serve to boost an individual's sense of competence, thereby increasing confidence in their ability to successfully perform the task. At other times, esteem support can be invaluable as it helps an individual remain confident and motivated when their skills are not improving as quickly as they might like. One participant described how believing our assurances that his golf would eventually improve was helpful:

> ...getting that confidence, just giving it time, and obviously like you said it'll gradually come. So when you actually do it like on here I suppose it came in one piece. It all came together. It worked out OK. I'm pleased with that.

Receiving esteem support can in itself directly bring personal pleasure or sense of pride. We have observed this on numerous instances, as the following excerpts from our field notes illustrate:

> Richard's face brightened when I talked about him looking athletic on the golf course, he seemed really pleased to have positive input about how he had played. He smiled a lot when I gave him encouragement and said a very warm 'thank you'. (Kitrina, 25 June)

> On the 3rd, following his tee shot, Andrew asked Julian 'Am I improving?' and was visibly pleased when both Julian and I enthusiastically replied 'Yes!' On the green, I asked him to make a shorter, slower swing and, taking the ball away, asked him to make a practice swing. 'Perfect! Now do the same swing again when I replace the ball' was my advice. That is exactly what Andrew did and, from 9–10 feet off the hole, the ball rolled straight in. 'Yesssss! Great shot!' was the general reaction from the group ... Andrew's reaction was fantastic: he visibly tensed, clenching his fists, rising taller by three inches, and grinning a huge beam. (David, 18 June)

While documenting the effects of esteem support offered by staff members, the second excerpt also hints at a potentially significant exchange, or sharing, of esteem support *between* participants. An exercise leader described how an unexpected exchange of esteem support occurred between two members of the golf group:

> The following day after the second session we went swimming with Ali and he met Jerry in the changing room and first thing he said, out clearly and precise, 'cause Ali mutters and is really hard to understand sometimes: 'Jerry! You're the one who hit the 170 yard shot! That was a fantastic shot!' Like that, so precise and so clear. He looked at the person and said it and it was absolutely amazing. And then he just went like that *[mimes dropping head to look at floor]*, he turned around to his locker and was all quiet again ... I've never seen Ali speak so clearly and so precise as that. Before that he would mutter and he probably wouldn't speak to Jerry so precisely like that 'cause he hardly knew him.

This excerpt documents an example of what to us is a mutual giving and receiving of reinforcement and support. That is, it is not only that individuals benefit from being the *recipients* of esteem support, but that they may also *give* esteem support to others through positive comments or exchanges. Like informational support, when the exercise leader recognises the potential of group members in this regard, their input to the esteem of others can also become a valued aspect of the activity and encouraged.

Emotional support

Emotional support is described as 'the ability to turn to others for comfort and security during times of stress, leading the person to feel that he or she is cared for by others' (Rees *et al.*, 2003, p. 137). Participants in our research have often talked about how emotional support – usually from family and friends and sometimes in the context of sport and exercise activities – has been important to them. One described the support he receives from his parents when he competes in races: 'My dad was there like. My parents used to go, parents go with me too on all these runs, they go with me and sort of cheer me on at the end.' In the words of another:

> Family as well, friends, they supported me since I was ill really ... used to come round, make sure I was up or I went out with them they asked how I was. You know just good friends really... Yeah. Yeah. Just care, care, care like. Care.

Alongside emotional support being provided by outsiders, we also observed that emotional support, like esteem and informational support, was at times shared *between* members of exercise and sport groups. In this way, participants both received and gave emotional support to each other through sport or physical activity and, as the following excerpt suggests, these steps can be taken without the session leaders being involved:

> Badminton has been a good place to meet people without necessarily having to sit and have a full conversation, particularly when you first start the group and are very nervous. It's nice that some of us meet afterwards for coffee etc. ... in the leisure centre cafe. Again there's no pressure to stay ... no one is expected to stay for a drink, but everyone is welcome to. That is something we do generally without the

coaches being involved, so again it helps us build friendships and a time to chat if we want to.

We were also aware that quite often, participants would suggest that the sport group provided something they had not experienced before:

Well I'm sort of supported. I feel supported with other people there yeah. It's people that I know mainly, especially the football team, its people that I never knew before but I got friendly with, made good friends, and we all just participated in sport . . . This is why I still come to [name of day centre] 'cause of the sports activities and what have you. I think it's important to keep it going.

While being difficult to document, time and again we witnessed subtle processes of mutual interpersonal emotional support taking place within the context of some sport groups which served to help bind group members together and, we suggest, create a sense of community. Intrinsic to this sense of community was group members' willingness to give and accept emotional support to and from each other. The following excerpt from our field notes provides an example of this process in action as several group members respond to photos one participant took of a previous week's golf session:

As we sat around waiting for the mini bus to be organised Peter said he had brought his photos. I was thrilled and asked to see them. He had gone to the trouble of getting a set done for us. The photos were of the group playing on the first week out on the golf course. I looked at them and wished we could use them. I passed them on to others who were interested. Jerry looked at them and particularly looked at photos of himself. He said that he needed to lose some weight. The words were said without withdrawing or looking overly concerned. Then he said, 'I need to come off of medication.' The others sat around were listening. Peter agreed, he said he had reduced or come off his medication then he said, 'I keep some just in case like.' Andrew had been listening too, he joined in affirming what the others had said, 'I keep some just in case too.' (Kitrina, 16 July)

This account shows the dynamic and complex nature of social support systems and particularly the delicate and unpredictable nature of emotional support. If one participant hadn't been enthusiastic about documenting the activity, the photos would not have been taken. If he had not wanted to share them with the group, or the group had been unavailable, they would not have been shared communally. If they had not have been shared, there would have been no spontaneous opportunity or catalyst for the group to comment and encourage each other about a concern that was relevant to them all. We suggest that at times like these, when individuals engage with and support each other in talking about shared personal issues, a valuable exchange of emotional support takes place. On this occasion it was made possible through participation in a sport group.

Reflections

As Corrigan and Phelan (2004) suggest, social support is a multifaceted and complex construct. We have attempted to shed some light on this complexity by considering how and when four specific dimensions of social support have been manifest in our own research. In keeping with the ethos of interpretive research, we aim to *illuminate* rather than *finalise* the ways in which social support processes operate in the context of exercise and serious mental illness. There are alternative perspectives and frameworks for considering social support. In recognition of this, we would like now to reflect on the ways in which this particular model relates to explorations of social support in other physical activity and mental health research.

In their study of a pioneering community gym for people with mental health problems, Raine and colleagues (2002) identify five qualities of effective gym staff. They describe these as the ability and willingness to:

- provide skilled fitness instruction
- offer personal encouragement
- monitor individual progress
- give practical support
- offer emotional support.

For us, these qualities revolve around an individual's ability to provide varied forms of social support and highlight the need for exercise leaders to be multiskilled and to take seriously their own role facilitating exercise participation. While qualities like these would ideally be present in *any* exercise leader, coach or personal trainer, we suggest that they are *particularly* important in mental health contexts given the complex support needs which may be present. As Crone and colleagues (2005) observe, it is likely that exercise leaders will need to draw on both professional skills *and* personal qualities in order to provide the most effective support.

While considering separate dimensions of social support provides insights into how provision can be more effectively made, it risks suggesting that each form of support is discrete or separate from the others. This has not been the case in our experience. Instead, we found that more than one type of social support generally occurred in combination. For example, three stages of intensive social support provision have been identified in the context of physical activity and mental health (Carless, 2007):

- *Awareness raising* – a preliminary social support strategy where the potential benefits of physical activity are highlighted;
- *Engagement* – during which time a form of exercise is identified which suits the personal needs and appeals to the interests of the individual;
- *Practical facilitation* – which often involves a long-term commitment to the organisation of physical activities alongside offering a combination of encouragement, direction, motivation, and reassurance.

We suggest that while informational support tends to dominate the first stage of awareness raising, engagement can best be characterised by a combination of both informational and esteem support. Practical facilitation, we suggest, is very often a combination of all four types of support in a dynamic process which is sensitive to the particular needs of the individual.

An excerpt from an interview with one exercise leader relays a sense of the dynamic process of social support provision in action. This excerpt focuses on the process of supporting initial exercise involvement:

David: So once you've had an idea of someone, how do you approach it, how do you broach the subject with them?
Just basically ask if they're interested really. It's either a yes or no. And then –
David: Really? As simple as that?
Yeah. Maybe they just think about it and then over time they ask us if they can.
David: You don't consciously, don't deliberately sell it to them then as being a good thing?
Yeah, but we're low input. We don't want to push it 'cause we don't want to, well I never do push them 'cause they usually back off sort of thing. They don't want to be put too much under pressure. The way I put it is just, oh, 'You'll meet people,' or 'Your mate comes along,' you know, like if you know they get on with somebody they buddy up sort of thing and um, yeah, I just, and fresh air and learn something new. But I don't really 'high pitch' it 'cause they're bound to back off, a lot of people back off.
David: OK, so there's a threat generally with this client group that if you come on too strong you're going to turn them off it and drive them away?
Yeah. They just feel pressurised a bit. And then it's got to be their decision ... So I think the best approach I always find is just gently bring it up and ask a few times, 'Have you thought any more about the golf?' sort of like, you know?
David: Yeah OK, so a sensitive, friendly, type of 'matey' approach almost?
Yeah, exactly. It's not, it's not going to be over-judged on it, it's not going to be part of their care plan or something like, it's going to be a gathering of people for a good golfing, a good session to do basically ... I just put it to them basically, make the suggestion, 'Hey! It's going to be good fun!' But at the end of the day it's down to them.

As this excerpt reveals, a high level of sensitivity to the needs of the individual, combined with a respect for individual autonomy and choice, is likely to be critical to the effective and ethical provision of social support.

One point of particular interest which has emerged in our work is the way in which individuals both *receive* and *give* social support *for* and *through* physical activity and sport. This sharing of social support, for us, has two implications. First, as Crone and colleagues (2005) have observed, it implies that individuals are able to draw potentially valuable support from not only mental health professionals but also other members of the exercise group. Second, while social support research has tended to focus on what individuals need to *receive* in terms of social support (e.g. Rees *et al.*, 2003; Corrigan & Phelan, 2004; Davidson *et al.*, 2005; McDevitt *et al.*, 2006), there is also, we suggest, a need to consider what participants are able to *give* to others in support terms. For us this point is particularly noteworthy as, according to Deegan (1988), the opportunity to give is in itself important in recovery terms. Deegan draws parallels between the experiences of people with mental health problems and people with physical disabilities to emphasise the importance of recognising:

the gift that disabled people have to give to each other. This gift is their hope, strength and experience as lived in the recovery process. In this sense, disabled persons can become role models for each other. During the dark night of anguish and despair when disabled persons live without hope, the presence of other recovering persons can challenge that despair through example. (p. 18)

Frank (1995) argues that giving, through acts of generosity to others, be recognised as an ethical responsibility of living with serious illness. For him, while ill persons may share what they have learnt through their experience of illness with another *for the benefit of the other*, something about the act of giving in this way also provides personal enrichment. One possible and significant benefit might be an enhanced sense of community. According to Deegan (1997, pp. 13–14):

community, *real community*, is not a place. It is not the place outside the institution. Community is not the buildings and streets that surround us out here. Community is not a place. Community is a way of being in relationship with one another.

With this point in mind, we ask whether the opportunity to provide social support *for* others, in the ways discussed here, might provide a valuable opportunity to experience real community through a different way of being in relationship with one another. This opportunity may in itself come to be seen as a valuable and life-enhancing experience by some people with mental health problems.

Key points

- Informational, tangible, esteem and emotional forms of social support are all likely to be beneficial when it comes to facilitating physical activity or sport participation in mental health contexts.
- Informational support (through one-to-one conversations) can be an effective way to raise an individual's awareness of why she or he might wish to commence a particular activity or sport. Later, information support (through effective teaching or coaching) can help increase knowledge and understanding of an activity resulting in sustained interest, motivation and success.
- Tangible support (in the form of transport, equipment, financial support) is often a prerequisite for sport and activity participation among people with serious mental health difficulties.
- Esteem support (through verbal persuasion and 'being there') can help increase an individual's confidence and self-efficacy for an activity or task. Some people with mental health difficulties depend heavily on this type of support, particularly during the early stages of participation.
- Emotional support (through a sense of being cared for) is important to many people and often depends on a broader social network of family and/or friends. Its presence relates to a sense of community and inclusion.
- While these different types of social support are very often a prerequisite *for* exercise participation, they can also be potentially beneficial outcomes which arise *through* involvement in sport and exercise groups.

■   Social support in the context of mental health is not a 'one-way street' – it is not only the case that people with mental health problems benefit from *receiving* social support but that at times they can also benefit from *giving* social support to others through shared membership of an exercise or sport group. This sharing process may be a valuable way of rebuilding a sense of community among people who are living with and recovering from serious mental health difficulties and is therefore worth developing and nurturing in physical activity and sport contexts.

Practitioner perspectives

10

Throughout the book we have attempted to provide information that will be useful for those who are interested in making physical activity or sport provision – of one form or another – within mental health contexts. This chapter fits with this same aim, although our approach here is different to previous chapters.

Over the past ten years we have come to know and work with several individuals who, in varying roles, have worked within physical activity and mental health. The research described in this book has benefited from their practice and experience. In this chapter we turn our focus onto the experience of three particular practitioners whose work, we think, illuminates, complements, enriches and develops the material we have presented so far. While there are now a good number of practitioners working in this field, we asked these particular individuals to share their experiences in part because of our personal knowledge and/or experience of their work and in part because between them they cover a wide variety of backgrounds and professional disciplines, settings (National Health Service and independent) and activities (sport, physical activity, outdoor activity, dance). In what follows, we present a brief biography of each person and then an interview with each of them which focuses on their own experience and perspective on practice and provision in the context of mental health.

Margot Hodgson

Margot Hodgson is a senior physiotherapist with Avon and Wiltshire Mental Health Partnership NHS Trust in Bristol, UK.[1] She has been one of the driving forces behind the Bristol Active Life Project (BALP), a physical activity and sport intervention aimed at

---

[1] Margot Hodgson can be contacted via email (margot.hodgson@awp.nhs.uk).

individuals with serious mental illness. It was funded by the Football Foundation which made it possible to provide a variety of sports and activities (football, badminton/table tennis, tennis, basketball, gym sessions, swimming and walking) at multiple community venues across Bristol. BALP has been one of the first projects in the UK to make sport provision for service users in the community and received national recognition for its achievements from the National Institute of Mental Health in England and was awarded the Positive Practice Award in 2005 for tackling physical health inequalities. We interviewed Margot in April 2009 about the project and about her involvement in physical activity, sport and mental health.

Kitrina: Margot, can you explain what your role is in the project and how you became involved in this groundbreaking initiative?

My role has evolved over the years. Initially, I was employed in a vocational unit to look at people's physical health needs and, through that, the project developed to setting up sport groups in the community for people with mental illness. I don't do so much 'hands-on' stuff now, but initially I went out with the groups and helped run the session. The project is at the stage now and has grown so that we have been able to employ people with the appropriate skills to fill those roles. My role now is liaising with the local council, overseeing the project within the Avon and Wiltshire Partnership and exploring ways to develop the project.

Kitrina: How long ago did you become a physiotherapist?

About thirty years ago, but I've been working in mental health for about fifteen years now. It started with me becoming aware how poor people's fitness levels were. You know, youngish men in their 30s getting out of breath just walking up a flight of stairs. So, that got me thinking 'How can we get people to be more active?' The first step was getting an exercise bike and a rowing machine, which was paid for by the League of Friends. I was working at Colston Fort [a rehabilitation day centre for people with severe and enduring mental health problems] at the time and there were no facilities for exercise so I got moved around every room in the place with that equipment, but it meant people could exercise two or three times a week. A problem at the time, and I still think it's a problem, is that people only wanted to do five minutes on the bike. If they go to a gym you have to pay membership or an entry fee, and so on. If you have to go through all that for five minutes it is not feasible. But that small start was really successful and showed there was potential. So then we set up a badminton and football group. Initially myself and the physiotherapy technician led the sessions. The first difficulty we faced was hiring a sport facility, which was immediately a challenge because there was no money in the budget. Fortunately, I had a sympathetic manager who liked football so he actually paid for us to have one indoor football session a week, and that was really successful.

Kitrina: Was it difficult at first to get people to try the bike and to get them involved?

Yes it was. I think it was something people thought they couldn't do. So it was very much a case of saying 'Just come and have a go,' 'See how much you can do,' 'Just do a minute, see how you get on,' very gradual. I was working in rehabilitation at the time, which is where the people with most need are, and I thought if we are able to get these people to do some exercise, and if it does work with this client group, who are the most difficult to engage, then it has the potential to work with everybody really.

Kitrina: What was the next step?

It was through one of the service users who was very keen to play in the Bristol Pro 5 [a 5-a-side football league] so he, with an occupational therapist, started to look at funding opportunities. They wrote to lots of businesses in Bristol and managed to get £500 from an insurance company to pay for a team of service users to take part in the Pro 5. So that was our first bit of funding!

Kitrina: What about restrictions, because alongside the activity, are a certain number of mental health staff required?

With all the sports groups which run in the community there has to be two mental health staff and that was difficult because there was only myself, who works part time, and a physiotherapist technician. But some of the occupational technicians were quite keen on football, so we managed to get their support to help with the groups. Then, with that being successful, we came to the conclusion that there must be funding out there for sport and disability. Then, that same service user brought information in about the Football Foundation. In the meantime we had actually got some funding from Sport For All, and I think that was £5000 for sport groups in the community, so that was used to set up three football groups.

Kitrina: Was service user involvement important at the beginning?

Absolutely and particularly that one chap, he was the one that was identifying funds and was working with the occupational therapist writing letters. When he brought in the information about the Football Foundation that was when we started to think, well, we do tick all the boxes. Working within the health service, however, we have restraints which mean we can't apply for outside funding, but the service users can.

Kitrina: That's complicated!

Yes, that is complicated, but these are just things that make it difficult. Over the years we had been meeting people from Bristol City Council and they were keen to work with us. Up to that point we never really managed to bridge the gap for how we could work together. When the Football Foundation funding opportunity arose they said they would hold the money in the City Council. In a way, that was the way forward, which actually was perfect because they could set up any number of groups you know for people with disabilities but our people could never access them. Within the mental health service, referrals are through care co-ordinators, so we can provide the right support for people to go to the groups. The big change was with funding we could also employ a qualified sport coach to run the session, because up to then it was the mental health staff. So then we started to take the exercise out of the mental health service to be more 'normal' and mainstream. But, of course, we also worked alongside the coaches so we have mental health staff in all the sports groups as well. The role of the council is to hold the funding, manage the budget, they employ the sports coaches and we manage all the referrals within AWP to make sure there is liaison with the coaches.

Kitrina: What advice would you give someone taking up an activity now?

Initially I would just have a chat, find out if they are interested in doing any physical activity and would describe some of the benefits, you know, 'If you go for a five minute walk you feel better.' I always provide something that is achievable, so going back to the exercise bike, I'd say 'Just try two minutes' initially, something he or she can achieve. Because often people think, 'Oh, I'm not sporty' or 'I can't play badminton' or 'Oh! I haven't played football since I was at school and I was never picked for the team.' So it is very much, or the tack I take is, 'It's fun, you'll meet new people, just go along and play for a bit, have a rest when you want to, go and see how you find it.' I remember one chap and so many times I said to him just to go along. Years later he's there every week and he loves it. But for a long time it was, 'No, no, no.' And now all his mates are there. So I always keep it low key, no pressure. But obviously it depends on the individual, some people you can cajole a bit and encourage where somebody else you say it once and that's enough. So I don't think there is a standard way that everybody responds. Individuals respond differently. I think to make sure the individual knows it is not a threatening situation, that they can go and find out what it's all about, then they can make their decision about whether they want to go back again. It's not saying 'If you go once you have to go every week,' but rather 'Go, you might like it' or 'You might not, but at least you have given it a go.'

Kitrina: What about other professionals coming into this environment, what would you say to them, reflecting on your experiences and what you have learned over the years?

Well, I think there are different schools of thought within the team, the staff team, which is good because we all have different backgrounds. As a 'non-sport-person' I very much come from the angle of, well, it's the taking part, it's the having fun, whereas I know for some people, they are much more focused on winning, and they do want their team to win, and so, I think, it is important to offer a spectrum, groups where people just have a kick around, and if there are people who are more competitive, and some of the footballers who play love the competitiveness of it, and winning the trophies and they should be supported to do that as well. So it's important not to put anybody in a box but rather work towards what they want to get from the groups. I think within most groups, another example is the badminton, some people just come for a knock around and other people are really quite competitive and they want a really hard game so, going back to what we were saying before, it's the skill of the coach or session leader working with the individual that makes both possible.

Kitrina: What advice would you give to coaches? Do you see them as a group that understand the needs of diverse individuals or do you think they have a lot to learn?

I think they have a lot to bring to the group because obviously they have a lot of skills within the area of sport and I think that's fantastic for our service users – they are highly qualified professionals and are good at their sport. But a large part of working with this client group is being able to engage them initially, and some are very frightened and apprehensive about going to a group so part of the job of the coach is enabling them to feel comfortable, to go at a level they can manage so that they don't feel threatened or undermined, that someone on the other court is doing better than them. Coaches need to ensure that whatever level people want to work at, it is right for them. Coaches also need to recognise the huge social side to it, because often people are very isolated. In my experience, other members of the team become their mates and that is a hugely beneficial part of going.

Kitrina: Looking back, what are the most difficult challenges you have faced?

The initial challenge was the facility hire and then the employment of sport coaches. Getting it to work as a whole has been challenging because everything is outside of the NHS, if you like. Our clients live in the community so they should have access to community facilities so our challenge has been to bridge that and we have been fortunate that we have developed a good working relationship with Bristol City Council. But this partnership hasn't been easy. We are a huge organisation and they are a huge organisation and we are coming from very different starting points. We are obviously health and clinical and they are more promoting, organising and administering sport. So the challenge is for them to understand our point of view and for us to understand their point of view. For us to understand their objectives and ways of working has required good communication and all the way through it's been a case of 'let's try this' and sometimes it works and sometimes it doesn't work and we have to go off at a different tangent. So things haven't been straightforward but we have tried to find a way to move forward. At the moment we are dependent on care co-ordinators to refer people onto the project, which is a bit frustrating. At Colston Fort I had direct contact with the clients and I would talk to anybody, they didn't have to look remotely sporty, and I would ask them if they fancied joining in. Whereas now, I wonder if care co-ordinators sometimes just think 'That person wouldn't be interested' – whereas, quite probably, that person might be interested. So, to address this issue now, we are planning on giving presentations to the community teams and talking about physical activity in order to encourage them to refer and engage people in these sessions. At the moment when someone is referred to the project they are supported by their care worker for the first two sessions, ideally. And then if someone hasn't gone for a couple of weeks we will phone them. Another issue is transport, you know, some people can't use public transport, so we are dependent on the care co-ordinators to address that issue, we can't organise and supply transport because we haven't enough staff to do that. But the groups are subsidised, so I think that covers that issue.

Kitrina: And they are city-wide?

Yes, so people can access activities near them, supposedly. Of course it depends on the sport. At the moment we have only one tennis group and one basketball group so that's not ideal, but it is a start.

Kitrina: Looking to the future, how do you hope to develop the project? You now have qualified coaches leading sessions and some of those individuals who are your clients have become coaches and led sessions. That's a huge step forward.

In the initial bid we wanted to offer an opportunity for those who were interested to take coaching qualifications. The aim was that some service users could possibly be employed as sport coaches or gain work experience. Another aim was to work with the voluntary sector as well as the council, all working together and everyone could access the group. But in reality that didn't work. We were the driving force but the council didn't have the resources or the understanding of how mental health service works, so although we tried to forge links with the voluntary sector we didn't manage to make progress. So, we worked on what we could do, which was working within AWP and working with the council. What was going to happen, the idea was that all the groups were going to be 'open' so that the sessions could be accessed by AWP and the voluntary sector. But what we have decided to do now is keep some groups 'closed' for those who are referred from AWP and they will have a sports coach and a member of staff from AWP. Then there are going to be open groups, which can be accessed by the voluntary groups, and these will be run by the coach without a member of the AWP staff. From our perspective, the open groups will be looked on as move-on groups. Some people might go directly into those groups, but we have people who are at the more unwell end whereas the voluntary sector are likely to have people who have been discharged. Though, funnily enough having said that, they have quite a lot of people in our groups so they straddle the two groups.

Kitrina: Some coaches are worried about an 'incident' working with people from a mental health service. How have you got round that?

I don't think anything major has ever happened in any of the groups I've organised. Commonly, people are anxious and need reassurance. It's difficult for me to sort out what someone may call 'an incident' and what is normal working with this group. Maybe a lot of the coaches are influenced by negative media portrayals of people with mental illnesses, whereas the biggest problem most face is they are frightened to go somewhere on their own. So in a way, the mental health support is there to help them get to a group and so on, not to influence their mental illness. But if there was an incident, it's in a public building and it's in the community and the coach or whoever would need to take appropriate steps just like with any other individual or group. But that hasn't happened. Most people are anxious going into a sport facility, imagining everyone will be in lycra, looking tanned and athletic, you know, I'd be nervous going to a sport facility! But it's not threatening once they have been and once it becomes familiar they are more likely to go again.

Kitrina: What have been the most encouraging aspects of BALP?

The driving force behind this, as I said at the beginning, was I noticed that people were unfit, so we got the exercise bike, got people doing a bit of exercise. But for me, it wasn't the fact that there were physical health improvements, but rather, that their mental health improved. And for some people, it was very marked. Initially, I was just trying to get them to do some exercise and then they came and did a couple of minutes on the bike. That built up to five minutes, then ten minutes, and with that, they just seemed more confident and then able to go along to the football groups. I think it was confidence and their self-esteem that was markedly different, and I suppose it was not focusing on mental illness. So when I saw them I'd say, 'How's the football?' and they'd go, 'Ahhh! We got five goals!' So they had something to get enthusiastic about. Again the social aspect was important, there were people to do things with, other people involved with thinking about developing the project, and they were empowered to look at things they could do to help themselves.

Kitrina: Do you think there are certain sports which facilitate those important experiences to be built up?

I think probably the football because immediately there is a team, they work together. But having said that the badminton group has been really successful, people come together, they encourage each other, you know if someone does a good shot, others are really enthusiastic and they are very inclusive, and will encourage people who are a bit hesitant, they look out for each other and have an empathy and support. The walking group which leaves from the library, and is run by two mental health staff, that's really good because there is time for people to talk. And I think the Pro 5, because it's out of the mental health system, that's really good.

Kitrina: That's great, Margot, is there anything else you think might be of interest to other people?

Well, it's beginning to be more widely recognised now, and even coming down from the government, which is encouraging and shows a change. But, from my position, the benefits are so huge, and for everybody. You know, perhaps for some it's really evident, but it's also cost effective and it's in the community. So I just think it's wonderful!

David Stacey

Since 1991 David Stacey has worked for the Community of St Anthony and St Elias in the southwest of England.[2] 'The Community' provides housing, support and rehabilitation for people with severe and enduring mental health problems and complex placement needs. As a member of the senior management team, David's responsibilities include co-ordinating a broad activity programme within The Community. We interviewed David about his work in June 2009.

Kitrina: What was your role when you first started 18 years ago?

I joined to develop an outdoor activities programme and my title then would have been 'outdoor activities manager'. Although we include other activities, we focused for 10, 14 years on developing outdoor activities.

Kitrina: Is that because that's something you're interested in?

Yes, I think I brought skills in that area. I trained as a teacher and one of my main subject areas was outdoor education and I used that background to develop the outdoor activity programme at The Community.

Kitrina: Did you have qualifications in those activities?

Yes, all the key ones. I was qualified to mountain leader standard, supervising rock climbing, coaching canoeing, so covering all the bases. There was a sense that the work The Community was doing involving adults with mental health problems in activities wasn't too common at the time. It was and still is a key part of the way the organisation functions. It is also to ensure that we are operating within the appropriate professional standards. One of the key things nationally at the time was the disaster at Lyme Bay where a routine canoeing trip for a group of youngsters developed into an incident which resulted in loss of life. That really brought the focus onto how outdoor activities are run and led to clear guidelines for under-18 provision. Though we work over-18, there was still a recognition that it was vital we should work within the frameworks of the national governing bodies. Also working in the area of mental health, some people might ask 'What are you doing taking people who are mentally ill to do adventurous activities?' That could be considered a risky thing to do. But really you've got to bite things off in manageable chunks and work through things step by step. You work out why

---

[2] The Community of St Anthony and St Elias has been the subject of a research study (Owens, 2004) which provides further information on the ethos and work which takes place there. David Stacey can be contacted via email (dstacey@comae.org.uk).

you're doing them and then you ensure that the framework you are operating in is all there. Part of that is safety and the competence of people leading the groups. If those things are in place you've got a sound professional framework for doing things, whoever you are working with.

David: You mentioned then about knowing why you are doing things, what were your reasons for bringing outdoor activity into the programme?

One of the core elements of The Community's work is to have a non-institutional environment, to take people who have had periods of being really ill – maybe needing secure psychiatric accommodation – but who have reached a phase where their illness is well managed. Perhaps they have been through that particularly tough time in their life and they are more settled and stable so you can look at them moving on and living outside a hospital or other contained surroundings. So a key thing people notice when they come to us is a real shift from an institutional care environment to a domestic living environment – ordinary houses, ordinary homes, like you and I might live in. That is the first foundation for any activity work that takes place. On top of that, by living domestically you are sharing a home with other people, rubbing shoulders with them, going through ups and downs of a day, sometimes you're happy with them, sometimes you're not. You've got to work that out and that can be a big step. Once that is going OK, what do you do with the middle part of the day? A lot of people go to work. The activities came in because people were perhaps not able to take the step into employment so there was this time which needed to be used. The other aspect relates to people's life experiences which, with the group we have, can be pretty tragic at times. They may have areas of their life when they were developing that are really not there or they may not have tried certain things at all. So the activities were a way of doing something different which people may not have tried before. Another aspect was to have fun and enjoyment. If these things could be fun and enjoyable that is a pretty good motivation for giving them a go. And a final aspect was physical fitness, being a bit more active. Perhaps people have had times where this hasn't been a priority and just to get out and have a sense that they can get out, do things, move around, build a bit of fitness, feel good about ourselves, our bodies – without focusing on those things but just going out and doing things – that was another element as well.

David: So it sounds like it's about being a person in all its fullness, as opposed to treating symptoms of distress?

Yes, absolutely. The ethos of what we do is that it is not problem-focused – it's not focused on illness. The Community is not a medical organisation – although a support network is there if it is needed. We are trying to create an opportunity for people to live an ordinary life given that some people's backgrounds and circumstances are a little bit extraordinary.

Kitrina: You mentioned the support network before you do activities, how important is that?

I think it's very important. My role with activities rests on a lot of other work that is done within the homes. You're working within a bigger team. For example, say you are planning a camping trip you're taking staff who know the residents really well so even though somebody in charge might lead the activity itself the support is provided by a group.

David: What kinds of things are you looking for in people in terms of development?

Often people are meeting activities for the first time – I often describe it like they are walking into a field of freshly fallen snow. There are no foot markers for them, there's nothing there. They just have this new area to explore and hopefully you can provide the support they need to go and explore it and see where they get with it. They may not tell you about this, they may need to because you'll see how they are at the end. I'd hope they develop some new skills, build a bit of confidence, realise they can do things they didn't think they could do before. One of the things the outdoor side is very useful for in mental health is how people cope with situations. They may come with a whole load of ways of coping from their past life but faced with a rapid on a river or a rock face, you can see them sometimes trying to cope in old ways but it doesn't work. So they have to look at a new way. But this is all going on quietly as they are faced with the very practical situation they are in. And the support we give is all about saying 'You can do this,' even if you're not saying it in that explicit language, you're doing it in other ways. You're opening up a little window. The surfing sessions are an example of an activity which started because of one resident who came to live with us who had in his past been a surfer. We asked if he'd like to go again and he said he would, but we weren't sure how it would go. So we went off with a surf school in north Devon, with an experienced staff team including a couple who were reasonable surfers, and two or three other residents who wanted to go, and everyone got in the water. But the resident who was the experienced surfer, he just headed off for the big waves out the back! Everyone else was happy to learn on the beginning waves but no, he just clicked straight into how he had been. One of the experienced staff members paddled out with him and he just surfed a bit further out, more independently, and started to pick his skills up again. The point about this is that although we had staff who are surfers, he almost left them behind because of his ability to get out to waves. So we realised we had to have a second instructor to buddy up with him and we were able to build from there. Going on from there, our surf sessions have become a regular, established trip because other people in The Community have really taken a shine to surfing and we now have a session each month for 10 months of the year. One or two residents have bought their own equipment. One of them has moved on to live independently but he still links with The Community for the surfing sessions. It's generated its own life.

David: It sounds like what you have set up has been very responsive to what individuals need in terms of the details of the activity?

That's an important part I think. Say for a surfing session, we'd go to a reputable provider and book a two-hour session. It may not mean that everyone is in the water for two hours – it may be that you have to gear the session such that Fred is going to come along and try this week but he may only spend half an hour in the water. But then, OK, when he goes and sits on the beach what are we going to do then? How will we manage that? We make sure that we plan for that so that someone goes and sits with him. It may be that he doesn't come back in the water or if somebody goes and chats for 10 minutes he'll come back in. We don't know.

Kitrina: These were big successes but what was the biggest obstacle you faced in the early years? Like you said, you had the skills but this had never been done before.

No big thing stands out. It was an advantage that I arrived [in post] at the end of the summer so the best outdoor months of the year were over. I spent time over the winter working as a 'house parent' within the houses so I got a real sense of what was happening and got to know people.

Kitrina: How many people would there have been then?

There were six homes and over 20 people. That period gave me a sense of the foundations of The Community's work and time to plan over the winter before getting going with the activities. I had really good backing in terms of getting the equipment we needed and a key thing was finding a vehicle. That was important because we had to transport people around and it wasn't going to be a car. But equally we didn't want to go the route of a minibus that looked institutional, that maybe had a name down the side. It just didn't fit, it didn't seem right. So we looked for a long-wheelbase Land Rover with 10 or 12 seats and we found one – at a budget – and that became our first vehicle. There was a sense that when you are going out to do something adventurous, as soon as you set foot in the vehicle it said something. You were there in this big meaty four-wheel drive, a big roof rack, and you were off somewhere! And you were slightly looking down at other vehicles on the road!

David: It was a turnaround.

Absolutely. Somehow you've shifted something even without saying anything.

Kitrina: When you started – 18 years ago – what activities did you run then? How has the programme changed over the years?

The programme was heavily based around outdoor activities. There was moorland walking, coastal walking, climbing and abseiling, caving, horse riding, orienteering, canoeing, camping trips, expeditions away – anything from four nights to ten nights. Sometimes they might be quite goal-specific, like the Wye valley where we planned to canoe a certain distance. We also did conservation-type work, we've had a longstanding relationship with the National Trust at a local estate and we use their base camp accommodation where we have a deal that we stay there three or four nights but we do a day's conservation work, so you are putting something back into the local area. And the work experience side of conservation has been important. It's easy to forget that the people who come to us may not have had the opportunity, or even consider that they can do something positive for the local community. The very practical work on an estate – first, it has to be done to the standard the National Trust expects and second, you can see what you've done. Then there's the feedback and recognition from, say, a warden who – independent of us – says 'You've done a really good job there.' Sailing using a local sail training organisation became part of the programme about ten years ago and activities such as surfing started six to eight years ago. A regular indoor sports session also took place though that seemed to run its course and we let it lie fallow for a while. One of the difficulties of working in the context I'm in is that sometimes things have a natural life and you've got to recognise if it needs a rest. You've got to keep things fresh otherwise there's a risk of staleness, of sameness. The sports session restarted last year as a games session including, for example, Brazilian beach football.

Kitrina: What's that?

That's what I thought! Basically, it's three-a-side football with mini-goals and no goalie and you stick a ghetto-blaster on with Brazilian music! It changes into something different. The session also includes variations on volleyball using a huge ball as well as more usual activities such as badminton and basketball. We called it 'Games in the Park' and held it at the park last summer. Now we've taken it back indoors and booked a sports hall. And that seems to have gathered a bit of momentum with quite a few people attending. It originally was the idea of a staff member who has a range of sports activity skills and was happy to bring those to his work in The Community. We also have a monthly five-a-side football session linked with a local supported living centre.

Kitrina: And have there been any recent developments?

Our activity programme has reshaped over the last five or six years such that it is less focused on outdoor activities and has become a broader programme which includes an outdoor element, a sport element, a music element and a creative activities element. There is even a fifth element emerging this year which is to do with the thing that makes our organisation a community as opposed to a series of care homes that share an administrative structure.

Kitrina: Was that a conscious decision to be more community-focused?

I think it was because as we looked at the outdoor component, it was quite developed – we have a monthly programme that goes on right through the year. But there was a sense of 'Are we meeting the needs of the diverse people we had in The Community?' When we analysed it, some people, we felt, got an enormous amount out of the outdoor things but there was maybe 50% who weren't getting so much out of it. So we looked to bring in some other components. We have done some quite big trips, to give an example, we canoed 100 miles of the River Wye over six or seven days and people have climbed the three highest mountains in England, Scotland and Wales, we've cycled across Devon. There have been some big achievements. But there was a sense of 'Who's driving this?' Were we coming up with these ideas and then asking people to take part – and several would – or can we develop it in a way that we would include more people.

David: It seems like you have a person- rather than activity-focused approach which attempts to provide what individuals need as opposed to setting different activities against each other in terms of bidding for time and resources?

I suspect over the last four or five years we have reshaped it. Part of that is conscious, part of it is recognising that these things have a life of their own and you've got to be alert to where it starts to bubble up in one area and think that's good, let's just go with it. Looking at a cross-section across the 25 residents, at one end we have several who get an awful lot out of the activity programme, they'll be ringing up each month to book onto the activities they want to do. There'll be others who'll dip in, who have things they like to do. And there'll be one or two who we don't really see on the formal activity programme. But that's OK as long as we're aware of the bigger picture. As people do move on, they are going to be linking up with the local community and they're going to be involved in their own interests in the community – work, hobbies, education – and they may be busy with their own thing.

Kitrina: So once somebody has moved on they can still come back and join in?

Yes, absolutely. And we look for feedback about what people want to do. We have an annual questionnaire go out in the spring looking for feedback on the last year's activities and what people want for the forthcoming year.

David: What qualities would you look for, David, in an activity leader?
Firstly there's the competence to run whatever activity it is they are running.
Kitrina: Would you say that they need particular competencies to work in mental health?
No. If it was a session that needed a particular level of leadership or qualification then we'd make sure that was there. But I don't look for a specialism in mental health. A lot of the skills that you'd find in a good outdoor activity instructor working with a broad range of groups – leadership skills, being able to relate well to people – are great for mental health because you're looking at including people and building an ordinary relationship. It's the ordinariness of those interactions – within whatever it is you're doing – that is important. Within that is a sense of expectation – you're saying, 'It's alright, you're included in this, you can do it.' It's not saying you're a special group or that we've got to look at you in a certain way.
Kitrina: I don't know that is so in lots of sports because the focus on sport skills is based on the Olympic model of 'training' people to become really 'good'. That's the environment lots of coaches work in – they haven't necessarily gained the people skills you talk about as basic in outdoor activities. I wonder if there is a different ethos in outdoor activity compared to sport?
That is interesting, I wonder. I suppose one of the aspects is the reason you're doing it which then shapes how you relate to the people who are involved with it. I don't know if I can answer it specifically but I can give an example that might shed a bit of light. A lot of the way we run the activities is that the activities are a means to an end. But the fact that they do sometimes have an end or a goal is important. Say we're going for a day's canoeing on the estuary of the Dart. First, there's a group of people going, it won't be the same group that live in a house, it'll be mixed. You're all meeting at the activity store and immediately there's a whole load of social interaction going on – people who haven't seen each other for a while, people maybe a bit nervous asking questions about the day. There's preparing the equipment, travelling in the Land Rover to where we're going. When we get there it's: 'How do you wear a buoyancy aid?' or 'How do you do that?' There's all this stuff going on before we've even got on the water. Then you're doing the trip, having a packed lunch and people are finding it's really nice or actually it's tough because the wind is a real pain today. They are gaining something in learning how to canoe or stretching their skills but people hopefully come back having had a good day. But then it may build to where we set goals in particular things. Like, do you want to do white water canoeing? If you want to do that then we're going to have to focus your skills a bit more. Do you want to try a longer expedition? Then you're going to have to get a little bit fitter.
David: What I'm hearing from what you're saying David is, rather than trying to fit people to the activity and skills, you are prepared to change almost anything to fit the activity and skills to the person – we're going to stop canoeing because people don't want that at the moment and go walking instead.
Kitrina: Or instead of 11-a-side, we're going to have three-a-side, a small goal and put music on because it makes it more fun.
There are two angles to that – if I relate it to the more recent dilemmas in my work. There is that sense of adapting it, being responsive and working to the needs of people. Then there's that shift of when people do get interested and do get

motivated to go in a certain way. Then the goal becomes, well, if you do want to go there then that's what you might have to do to get there. It then becomes: 'Are you willing to make that little bit of extra commitment?' A simple example, if people are going to go on a moor walk they need to wear the appropriate clothing and a lot of that is to do with safety – we can't bend those rules and have to work within those boundaries. That's quite a key thing – some people say 'Why do I have to wear walking boots?' and you are immediately into an area of dialogue and discussion. But actually in the end, if you are going to walk, you do have to because it's down to safety.

David: Have you got any advice for others who are trying to start an activity opportunity in a mental health context?

Well, the overall thing is it's an incredibly valuable area. So many people get so much from the activities. In what I've said I've separated the mental health area, but this is ordinary things that lots of people do and get so much benefit from. Why should it be different for people with mental health problems? In a way I don't see myself working with people with mental health problems – I work with Samantha, Jane, Bill. It's just that what they have to cope with in their lives at the moment is this area called mental health. It's a valuable area because it comes with so many other things: the physical health side, the social interaction, doing something new, learning new skills – it's all part of life. If you can find a way in and people enjoy it then it's really important.

David: We're living in a culture that seems to be dominated by outcomes: for something to be set up – and certainly continued – we are asked to demonstrate that there are positive outcomes. What is your experience of that?

The client group we work with is very individual. If you look at the mental health professional's way of describing that client group, it's those with severe and enduring mental health problems and complex placement needs. That's quite a specialist group. So when it comes to evaluating the effectiveness of it we report to the authority that places a person with us, some of the evidence you would get to show that it's a valuable placement is that they are still with us. You may be looking at people with erratic placement histories who have not stayed in one place for any length of time. You would be looking at how they are participating within the home, within the local community but also the activity programme. So you would then say that a person has been walking and we may not perceive that as a major thing but for the referring authority it may be significant. And there's also the testimony of the individual – who might say 'I've been doing this, I've been doing that' – and the care team, the people who have known this individual over a longer period than we have will see what that person is like. So their evaluation will be based on that.

Kitrina: That's really important. You're not just looking at numbers – it's their particular journeys that you're looking at.

Yes. You're looking at a person. There's quantitative bits of a person – height, weight – but then there's the 'How do they walk in?' 'Have they got a spark in their eye?' 'Are they looking you in the eye when you're talking?' All sorts of things are going on.

Kitrina: This is important in terms of funding when people no longer join an activity. It's frequently seen that the activity is failing rather than it's done that person good and they're on to something else now. But it's looked at that unless you keep the numbers up it is failing.

I think that is such an important point. We have activities when you think 'Nobody's doing climbing anymore, what's gone wrong?' when actually the thing is to stand back, assess it a bit more maturely, and – it might be something wrong with the session that's putting people off – but more likely it has run its course for a while.

Kitrina: I can see that happening: an activity has provided a benefit and now the person needs something else.

Yes. There's a risk in the context I'm in of creating this bubble of these fantastic activities that's not really real. When people move on they're not going to get that outside. We may be able to pat ourselves on the back and say we've just taken a group of six severely mentally ill people and canoed across Scotland with them but we have to continually ask ourselves, 'Where does it leave them?'

Gerry Turvey

Gerry Turvey is a dance choreographer and facilitator of movement activity. She works with a range of community groups and professional companies as well as lecturing in dance at several universities. Much of her work is what she terms site-specific chore-ography, which entails creating dance and performance pieces for and in particular environments, locations and settings. Based in Leeds, UK, Gerry also works for the so-cial enterprise and charity organisation Hoot, based in Huddersfield, West Yorkshire, which offers opportunities for people to be involved in music, dance and other creative activities as a way of improving physical and emotional well-being.[3] We interviewed Gerry about her work in July 2009.

David: Tell me about your background in dance, Gerry.

I first trained as a visual artist and it wasn't until after I'd finished my art course that I went to a few dance classes and thought, actually, this is what I want to do. My body was calling! So I re-trained in France and Poland and London, in dance and physical theatre mainly, with people I wanted to work with who I felt could give me what I needed. And about once a year I'll do some further training with people I feel I can learn from. I did a two-year training with a dance company called Jabadao who work in the community, mainly with people with learning disabilities and older people, this was incredibly practical and really useful, and has been the basis of all my community work.

David: So those two years gave you the insight of seeing dance working for people?

Yes. I think it was the woman, Gay Parker, who ran most of the training– she was really inspirational. When I'm in a sticky moment I always think about her now. The way she worked with groups was so inclusive, so supportive and encouraging of whatever people offer.

---

[3] More information on Gerry Turvey's work is available at www.turveyworld.co.uk and she can be con-tacted via email (turveyworld2@yahoo.com). More information on dance specialists working in the UK is available from the Foundation for Community Dance (www.communitydance.org.uk). Information on the social enterprise and charity Hoot can be found on their website (www.hootmusic.co.uk).

David: Can you give me an example of how she might do that?

She might start a group – even a massive group – in a circle and ask each person to say their name and do a movement. People with severe physical disabilities may only move a finger, but that will be accepted and included and valued. That is the basis of the work. If you carry that through – that whatever people offer is valued – then you can move them on so the next day you say, 'Well, you did that yesterday, can you find something else?' It's encouraging people to find their own way through creative movements.

David: Dance and mental health is a new area in that very little has been written about it to date. I'm very interested to hear about your own background and work related to mental health.

I think dance saved my life really, in many ways. A lot of the reason I went into dance was because I wasn't comfortable in the world and I didn't know how to express that. So some kind of art form and the physicality of dance really suited me. I need that physicality. I know that it is valuable to me so I am motivated to share that with others. I suppose I have some understanding of what it is to be mentally ill because I've been there a little bit myself and I know other people who have too. So I come from an understanding of what mental ill-health is and I think that's quite helpful.

David: Can you tell me a little about the organisation you work for?

The organisation I work with is called Hoot and is one of only a few who work with mental health needs. They get referrals from community mental health teams, CPNs, GPs and hospitals and people self-refer as well. It started as a music organisation, definitely based in the arts, rather than therapy. And they, in the main, facilitate workshops in music – drumming, singing, guitar, they've got recording studios and they also do songwriting. They have their own premises and the dance has been going on there for quite a few years now and is becoming more embedded within the organisation.

David: You mentioned it's art, not therapy, what's the distinction there?

I don't really know what therapy is, I'm not a dance therapist. Whoever I work with, I come as an artist and share my art form and I'm very clear about that. I see the benefits of it – people grow and learn, get more confident and get in touch with their body – but I don't analyse people's movement. I try to tap into people's creativity and be very accepting of whatever they offer. We're doing art every week – we're just not necessarily showing it to the public, it's just within the group. And I like that, it's sort of excellence within a small space.

David: From that perspective – of creativity and being an artist – what are your goals for a dance or performance session?

I suppose it is that people come and feel satisfied, feel included, feel better when they leave than when they came, engage with each other – so there's some kind of interaction between people. And I think – it's not really a goal, it's a spin-off for me – I'm continually surprised in a really good way by what people do in the sessions. I'll set up a task and then people will do amazing things with that task.

David: So they take it beyond what you envisaged?

Yeah. I suppose that's the thing with creativity, particularly in mental health, people seem to be very creative and are often not afraid to share that. I suppose that's one of my goals, that people will feel 'able' – it's about what people can do and what they can offer. Again, it's about acceptance of what people offer, and not making people feel excluded in any way. Generally my classes bring people together to share their different body histories through experiencing, and appreciating moving together.

David: Can you tell me about what you do to create that kind of acceptance?

I might offer a movement task – maybe individual, or partner or small group – with no pressure to get anything 'right' unlike, perhaps, dance technique where you're aiming to get, say, extension in your leg or your arm. I offer an open task where people can put themselves physically into it in whatever way they choose. I will always encourage people to challenge themselves and go further but I will also always do so by drawing attention to the qualities of what they're doing.

David: So the tasks are not so much outcome-based?

No, it's process, it's very much process. It's often improvised work but the tasks are quite structured in a way that people can access – they're not scary tasks!

David: So the people you work with, what are they coming to you for?

Well, some of the people have worked with me before and like dancing. They call it 'Gerry-dancing' now apparently! People were going 'What's this called?' and one of the support workers said, 'I think its Gerry-dancing!' I suppose they come because they know they feel safe in that space, that it's a good space to come to. They know they can come and make a cup of tea and they can join in the session or they can sit out if they want to. They know that no-one is going to tell them what to do – they are allowed to just be. And hopefully people will get a little bit in touch with their body and their breath and interact physically with other people. They don't have to express themselves verbally – I don't know what anybody's issues are unless they choose to share that with me and most people haven't. It's just a group like any other group in a way.

David: That's interesting you saying it's just like any other group. Do you work differently with a referral group than you might with another group?

Not really, no. Perhaps there's a little bit more allowance for people to go and have a cigarette, although I try and discourage that, I try and say we're not going to have a break, we'll work for an hour and a half and then we'll stop. If people feel uncomfortable I say sit out if you need to. But then I'd say that in any group.

David: Do you have a philosophy or ethos that underpins your work?

Yes, I do, but I don't know how to even begin to put into words! It's a 'can do' attitude but it's also about excellence in the art form. It's about 'can do' but it's also about not dumbing down dance as an art form.

David: Is there a tension there?

No, I think if you approach it with integrity. Say for instance, you're doing tondues, which is extending the leg, and somebody can't move their leg, then you ask them maybe to do it with their arm. But you wouldn't accept a bent arm because that exercise is about extension – you go to the full extension you can manage. It's about challenging and making suggestions for improvement in a way that people can accept. Often the professional dance ethos is about beating people up and saying 'You must be better! You'll never be the best!' but that is definitely not my philosophy. But it is about pushing people a little bit, in a good way, because you can only grow by being challenged.

David: How do you make sure you are challenging people in a 'good way'?

I work visually a lot. I try to see what people offer and how they are during the session and at the end of the session. It has a lot to do with the way you say things, encourage, offer alternative suggestions.

David: I imagine it has a lot to do with knowing the individual to avoid pushing them too much or in a way they find damaging?

Yes. It goes back to my training with Jabadao which taught me that it is always a group of individuals in any class, it is not about 'a class' – every person in that class has a different need. And that philosophy applies to choreography too – if somebody can do a fantastic handstand, you're going to use that in the piece, and if somebody else can't then you won't. So you're kind of using people to their best, in a way.

David: That's a very co-operative way of working, you're trying to build something together with the best of what each person can bring.

Yes, and that's how I make choreography. I set tasks, see what people do with it and then refine and develop it.

David: I like the idea that whatever a person is able to bring can be incorporated in the performance. So they choreograph something they can actually do rather than someone else choreographing something that they might not be able to do. That to me is very significant because sometimes in sport there is a standard you must reach to be able to do something and some people can't reach that.

Yes, yes, so then you're on the scrap heap – you're not valid. In dance, even in a professional company, if a dancer gets injured you might have to adapt their part so they can do it in a different way or that someone else can do it.

David: Some coaches or activity leaders might be worried about an 'incident' when working in mental health settings. What has your experience been in relation to that?

I did have something, but you see it doesn't bother me, what people might call an 'incident', because I'm accepting of how people are. But there was one woman, quite disturbed, but she came to the session anyway. She was in and out of the group so I just let that happen. Then every so often she'd say something quite abusive verbally, which was a little bit disturbing for the rest of the group, but I try not to take stuff personally. But then I put on a piece of music and everyone was just waiting for the next task – there was no-one else in the space – and she just took the space and did her own amazing dance all across the space. Everyone just kind of looked at her and it was quite incredible. I always remember that because it so touched me. I thought really I shouldn't worry about trying to contain because the space is there for people and that's the point of this session, that the space is theirs.

David: That's a lovely example.

Most people can work with each other but there are sometimes people who don't want to be physically touched and we do a lot of physical contact. One woman said 'I don't want to do the contact stuff,' and I said 'That's OK, fine. Have a cup of tea during this exercise and then come back in and you can work with me.' So I suppose I do make more concessions in a mental health group in that sort of way because I know there can be issues like that for people. I think it's a bit magical what happens in the sessions, unplanned-for things when people suddenly do things which I hadn't asked them to do – it's like, 'Oh! Wow!'

David: *David Stacey was saying that too, about serendipity, things happening by chance and leading somewhere or developing unexpectedly. It points to a need to retain an openness within sessions.*

Yes, yes. Every week I am surprised at what people offer and what they can do. A lot of the way I approach the work starts with relaxing, working with the breath, sometimes lying on the floor for quite a while and just letting go a little bit. I think it's helpful in letting go of physical blocks – you hold a lot of tension in your body without even knowing it. Everyone's got their own pattern of hold, so you can start to work through that a little bit, breathing through different parts of the body.

David: *Is there an example from your work that you would characterise as successful that you could tell me about?*

Yes, the group I ran with Hoot for about a year on a Wednesday evening. It was an open group but a regular core of people came, rain or shine. We worked towards a performance for the opening of the building. It was 100% their work – I just shaped it.

David: *Were the people that came to that group dancers before?*

No, though some had touched on dance before, or done some yoga.

David: *So how did you help a group of beginners create a whole performance?*

Through structured tasks. For instance, I have one activity called 'Centre-never-empty.' The group forms a circle and there's always got to be one person in the centre doing something and then you just add on to it, everybody can come and go as they like, it's great improvisation and you get loads of really nice patterns and shapes happening, it has its own life. So that's an example of an easy-access task where you can choose to go in or not.

David: *So you're included whether or not you want to be in the middle?*

Yes, yes. Then you can develop that into a piece. And performance quality is important to me as well, I'll always work on that – how people perform. For some people with mental health issues that's a massive thing, to actually be performing, in terms of confidence, positive feedback, working as a team.

David: *What qualities does a dance specialist in mental health need do you think?*

I think you need to be really clear in your art form, confident in yourself as an artist and what you offer. It's about being there in the space, with the group, and being able to communicate what it is you want to share. If you can do that you can work with any group. The other thing, particularly in mental health, is flexibility. Being able to improvise – which is a big part of dance anyway – to think on your feet. I think one of my strong points is focus and I think that is an issue in mental health, there's this thing that people in mental health can't focus for more than five minutes and people let them do it. Whereas I would prefer to say, 'OK, we're going to focus for this hour now, this is what we're going to do.'

David: *So there's a sense of quality of engagement?*

Yes. It's also about being able to give the task clearly – being able to show it, demonstrate it – and find the right music that supports that task. It's knowing how long to let the task run and knowing how to move it on to the next stage, then also knowing how to give feedback to people and not be fazed by difference, being accepting of people in a positive way. A lot of people seem to have a lot of fear around mental health. That's one of my strengths, I'm not afraid of people.

David: What advice would you offer to somebody who is interested in using dance in a mental health context?

Well, get a skilled dance practitioner in, someone with experience of community dance work. Someone who has got some mental health awareness would be a positive thing. It's also important to provide a decent space – not to go into a day centre and do it there, the space is not given over to dance and it's a lot harder to get the group to focus. If they come to a dedicated space that is meant for dance, it's a different kind of space, plus it's neutral, it's for that purpose. I always have a support worker with me – personal support workers if necessary – we do the session together. So, for instance, if someone leaves the support worker can go out to talk to them and then we can de-brief afterwards which is really helpful. Mostly they just join in the group but if someone has got an issue then they are there.

David: One of the reasons why dance has captured my interest this past couple of years is the way that it combines physicality – fitness, strength, flexibility, which is important to me, I get pleasure from that – with creativity.

Yes, yes. I know I'll feel differently after doing a dance class to before. I'll feel more open, stronger and I'll have used all my muscles. You don't think about anything else for the time you're doing it – you can't, because you're concentrating so much. And I like that complete absorption, for that hour, in your body. I sort of get it a little bit from swimming but my mind drifts off when I'm swimming. In dance, I've actually got to focus on where my foot is and where the next step is.

Key points

- Most physical activity and sport groups start small – often with just a few participants doing light activity for a short period of time. This is a positive first step as (by and large) *any* participation or involvement is better than *none*.
- During the early stages of physical activity participation in particular, effective support is critical. Most people depend on support and encouragement of both a practical and psychological kind (see chapter 9).
- Programmes and opportunities tend to evolve and develop over time. Often this process is serendipitous – it depends on the occurrence of chance events. It is wise to be responsive to and allow for unexpected and unplanned developments and progression.
- Flexibility and responsiveness to the needs and aspirations of individuals at different points in time is key to developing programmes which are sustainable and beneficial.
- Activity and sport groups can sometimes be short-term endeavours. If attendance rates at a particular group dwindle this should not automatically be taken as a failure. Groups sometimes serve a useful function as a 'stepping stone' for individuals to move on to something else (see chapter 6). A degree of freshness and novelty may help retain the interests and meet the needs of long-term service users.
- Indicators of the value and benefits of activity and sport groups need to take a holistic and person-centred perspective. The absence of measurable quantitative

change does not imply that a programme is worthless. Attending to an individual's life journey – or life story – often provides valuable testimony of the personal benefits of activity involvement.

- A person-focused (as opposed to an activity- or skill-focused) ethos and orientation is critical, particularly during the early stages of participation. During this time, the activity needs to be tailored to suit the needs, preferences and abilities of the individual – rather than trying to fit the individual to a predetermined activity. As the individual becomes more confident, committed and proficient it may be appropriate to consider more closely the personal development that is necessary to achieve progression.

- We suggest that alternative forms of activity and sport are considered which may appeal to a wider cross-section of people. For example, dance – and other creatively oriented activities – is more likely to be appealing to some women and girls who are not interested in competitive sport.

11

A story from practice

[Stories] long to be used rather than analyzed, to be told and retold rather than
theorized and settled. And they promise the companionship of intimate detail
as a substitute for the loneliness of abstracted facts, touching readers where
they live and offering details that linger in the mind.

Arthur Bochner (1997, p. 434)

Having almost reached the end of the book, we are aware that we have presented
much information and discussion relating to physical activity, sport and mental health.
Paradoxically, we are also aware that there remains so much we have *not* been able to
say. While one reason for this is practical (a book can only include so much material!),
another reason has to do with our primary reliance so far on data gathered through
interviews and conversations.

In any social setting, so much takes place beyond the realm of explicit verbal interactions, as many potentially important events or phenomena go unspoken. This
is certainly true during sport and physical activity sessions in mental health settings.
While talking to participants through interviews and informal conversation offers us
many insights into their experiences, what we hear through these interactions can never
provide more than a partial picture. Some things relating the nature of individual experience will remain unexpressed, unspoken, 'hidden' in the margins. In the context of
mental health, sport and physical activity, we suspect that these kinds of phenomena
may be important for two reasons.

First, as Baldwin (2005) and Stone (2006) observe, some experiences relating to
mental distress can be impossible to put into story form. In other words, certain
experiences are not in themselves amenable to being *talked about* or *pinned down*
in the form of a 'tidy' interview or coherent conversation. Second, physical activity
and sport are fundamentally *embodied* practices – they depend upon expression and

involvement through bodily movement. As Sparkes (2009) points out, if we are to develop richer and more complex understandings of people's experiences in sport and exercise, it is necessary to consider alternative ways of gathering data which might be better suited to recording the nuances of embodied experiences. These approaches are likely to rely upon a broader range of senses (e.g. vision, hearing, touch, smell, taste, perception) than are typically utilised during research studies.

It is this kind of approach which we utilise now in an effort to explore and represent the lessons we learned through a golf programme (and an accompanying ethnographic research project, see Carless & Douglas, 2004) which we ran in the context of a day centre for people with severe and enduring mental health problems. By focusing on observational and experiential data (i.e. what we *experienced* and *observed* as researchers and practitioners), we want to provide a further perspective on physical activity, sport and mental health to complement and enrich the material we have presented so far. This approach – critically – has allowed us to include those events and phenomena which may have passed without remark, yet are nonetheless significant in the context of this topic.

The approach to representation which we use here may be considered a *confessional tale* (Van Maanen, 1988), which we choose in order to reveal *ourselves* (as researcher-practitioners) within the text. In a confessional tale, Sparkes (2002, p. 59) suggests, 'the ubiquitous, disembodied voice of the realist tale is replaced by the personal voice of the author, announcing, "Here I am. This is what happened to me and this is how I felt, reacted, and coped. Walk in my shoes for a while."' Making our own role explicit is important because, as we discussed in chapter 2, it brings *reflexivity* to our research accounts. Reflexivity – to point at ourselves (as researchers) pointing at our participants' lives – allows the reader to attend to the ways factors concerning the researchers themselves might influence (for example) the interpretations, conclusions and recommendations which are put forward (see Etherington, 2004).

We return to a storytelling approach in an effort to *evoke* rather than *explain* some of the insights, understandings and truths which were revealed to us through the weekly golf group. Writing a creative fiction (see Sparkes, 2002) offered us the best chance of achieving this aim because it allows the creation of scenes which, while not always staying true to the *facts,* stay true to the *experience.* Accordingly, the stories which result are not necessarily tied to real events or real people, but instead attempt to communicate how 'things *like these* happened to people *like these*' (Angrosino, 1998, p. 101). As Laurel Richardson (2000) points out, fictional writing is a dynamic creative practice, a method of analysis, enquiry, discovery and interpretation. Through creating stories, a writer/researcher is able to deepen her knowledge of human behaviour through stretching the limits of her imaginary visions. The writer documents, in her mind, the minute details of her characters, their movements and glances, as well as what they feel, hear, see, touch and imagine and then recreates them in order that others can see.

We offer the following fictionalised story – written by Kitrina and consisting of a series of interlinked scenes based on events which occurred during the weeks of the golf group – as a way to further explore the kind of significant experiences and phenomena which can occur in the context of physical activity, sport and mental health. We hope that through this story we may be able to voice some of the issues, lessons and difficulties which are not present in the preceding chapters, in a way that stimulates the understanding and thinking of other practitioners and researchers.

Scene 1: corridor in Hadden Vale [a mental health day centre], Thursday 12.45 pm

'Come on, Brian!' encouraged Amanda the physio. 'You'll enjoy golf, it's out in the open, it's going to be taught by a qualified golf pro. You used to play golf, didn't you?'

There was silence and no eye contact. Brian was thinking. A withered hand tightened around his breathing, a dark shadow approached, his body sucked out from the inside, he focused, looked hard at the table in front of him, and the darkness let loose its grip. He began thinking again: Who would be there? Where would they go?

'It won't cost you anything, the programme's been funded, and we start in here next Wednesday. We're going to use the gym down the road for the first week and do indoor putting, the following week we'll be going to a driving range, there's even a minibus been put on to take everyone.'

The hand tightened its grip again, the dark shadow closed in on him from behind. Brian focused on the table. Then he began to consider everything Amanda had said. How would they get to the gym? Who else would be there? What would they have to do? How long would it go on for? His stomach tightened, his breathing shortened, a cold death crept forward lurking behind his shoulder – he dare not turn round.

But Brian liked golf, his hero was Tiger Woods, he remembered long ago hitting the ball like the tiger ... he even had a golf ball at home somewhere and a few clubs in a cupboard. 'Yep, I'll play,' he said, after several moments of silence. A huge smile broke across Amanda's face. Four people had now agreed to sign up for the golf sessions.

Scene 2: Manor Vaults pub, Friday 6.15 pm

'You don't understand,' said Tom, slightly exasperated, protective of the people he'd been playing football and badminton with. 'What works with other golfers won't necessarily work here. You can't just come in and coach them like you would any other group. These people have severe and enduring mental illness – do you understand what that means? Schizophrenia, bipolar, most of them are on antipsychotic medication, have you seen the side effects of that? Some of them have been in an institution most of their lives, others have been in and out of care or sectioned ...' Tom stopped in his tracks. Was he becoming the very type of person he didn't want to be by describing the group he'd been working with in this way? As lead researcher of the project 'Exploring the mental health benefits of physical activity', his initial plan had been to measure the participants' psychological health through perhaps the feeling states questionnaire, the temperament and character inventory, the Beck depression inventory maybe, or the satisfaction with life scale. That idea had received short change from the consultant psychiatrist at the centre.

'Do you realise,' Professor Milbourne said quietly, removing his glasses and fixing his gaze on Tom, 'the people you would like to understand have already filled in every questionnaire going, they have already been measured, tested, charted and categorised. I couldn't support you doing any more of that.' His head tilted slightly to the right and his body relaxed as if he'd heaved a sigh of relief. 'But, if you were to come in and spend time with them, maybe play sport with them, get to know them and their lives, you know, conduct some type of ethnographic research, maybe interviews, then I would give your proposal my full support and encourage the ethics committee to accept your research proposal.'

That meeting had been an important watershed for Tom. He understood then why he had felt some tensions with the grand plan for his PhD research which, while being completely acceptable in scientific terms, may well have posed problems for the participants and would most likely have ended up portraying them in a less than positive light. Being sensitive and aware, Tom already knew how researchers had in the past 'treated' – and mistreated – almost every population they had studied. He did not want to do likewise. He also knew from his own mental health experiences that there was a blurred line between those who think they are 'normal' and those who are categorised as 'mad'. The distance between the two, Tom knew, was closer than most people were prepared to admit. He felt uncomfortable talking and writing about *them* and *us* and presenting himself as the so-called 'expert'.

Having spent the best part of a year attending the day centre and joining in the football and badminton, Tom now felt protective towards these people who had become friends and with whom he had built good relationships – he had been sensitised to their problems and needs. He had also, through talking with Jessie, learnt that the group she was researching – elite athletes – shared a surprising number of similarities in terms of mental health with the group he was studying. Both he and Jessie were aware – and ashamed – of the contrasting ways people responded to the two groups. They saw how the press and fans responded to professional golfers with awe and respect and responded to 'mad people' with fear as the media hyped up stories of mental illness with hysteria and negativity. So on the one hand, while he thought there would be nothing better than to offer golf coaching to the group at Hadden Vale, he also realised that some of these individuals may be very different to the golfers Jessie had been used to coaching and, unlike her golfers, this group would not be so welcomed by club members with minds narrower than the fairways of their golf course. However, in pointing this out, was he becoming just like everyone else? Stereotyping his friends? Making assumptions about the problems they might face being coached? And making assumptions about how Jessie might coach the sessions?

His concerns were well placed. As an educator he had experienced the dark side of golf culture. During seminars to golf coaches, he had felt the stare of club secretaries simply because his hair touched his collar. He noticed eyebrows furrow at his untucked shirt and he had the indignity of once being asked to leave because he wasn't wearing a tie – until they realised this young man was Dr Swann, in the clubhouse to teach their club professional. He didn't want any of his friends to experience this type of small-minded pettiness, or experience any of the other elitist, sexist and able-bodyist attitudes that golf was renowned for. These concerns punctuated his thoughts as he tried to negotiate with Jessie what was the best strategy for the golf project. Tom wanted to be sure Jessie had thought all these issues through. He needed to know that she was aware of the problems and would be sensitive to the group's needs but, halfway through his speech, he realised that perhaps he was coming on a bit strong. Tom took a sip from his beer, replaced the glass carefully on the table and rotated it in his hand half a turn. Then, not taking his eyes off his pint, he continued.

'What I mean,' he said, this time more quietly, and taking a slow breath, trying to be a little less passionate, 'is that none of the other sessions are coached. People turn up, there's no pressure, we play football, it's not like boot camp with a sport coach barking instructions. I don't want ...' taking his eyes away from the beer he looked up at Jessie, 'I don't think it would be a good idea for you to do too much coaching. I don't think it will necessarily be what everyone wants.'

Jessie listened to everything Tom said and watched him intently. She too had been ashamed of the sport which earned her public fame, success and privilege. But she was also aware Tom hadn't seen her coaching, he wasn't aware of what her focus would be. She knew her focus would be the person, not the game, she knew how to bake cakes to share and she knew how to break the complicated swing down into little bite-size morsels so that anyone could understand and join in. Like Tom, Jessie had also been shaped by others who opened her eyes.

'Do you realise,' Dr Hicks had said, lecturing Jessie and the other first-year sport science students about disability in society, 'that when people in wheelchairs are, say, at the checkout at the supermarket, the person at the till is more likely to speak to whoever is pushing the wheelchair as opposed to the person in the chair? It's like they don't exist. Can you imagine what that's like? Have you ever thought about the lack of disability access to public spaces? What it says about our society? Have you thought about the sports *you* play? Do coaches prefer to teach elites? Do the kids with disability get a chance to join in? Or are they sent off for "special coaching"? Or worse, do they just have to just sit and watch?'

In one moment Jessie saw herself as just like the checkout staff. Could she really be so uncaring? So unaware? Vowing to try to see the person, not the disability, Jessie was self-aware enough to know that she had a lot to learn. The more she read the more she became aware. Those comments had been a catalyst for her to ask herself why there was so little interest in coaching people who fall outside the 'norm' and why golf was so exclusionary. She had dared to dream how it might be different.

Scene 3: café at Hadden Vale, Wednesday 12.40 pm (week 1)

Jessie arrived as Tom was introducing the group to plans for the coming weeks.

'This week we're going to have a putting game. On the floor of the gym we've marked out six bull's eyes around the room, and then around each one, a number of larger circles. Points are awarded based on how close you get to the centre.' Tom smiled at Jessie as she slipped in the back of the room, but continued without stopping. 'You will be playing as a team and so the game is to see how many points we can score. There's six putting holes and you'll probably have time to go round twice.'

It was the first time Jessie had been to the day centre. The room was cool in comparison with the warmth of the summer sun outside and its starkness reminded her of her school cafeteria with tables grouped together in formation. Scattered around the tables were a few empty mugs and biscuits sitting on plain green plates.

'We've got putters for everyone and Jessie will help you get the right grip, set up and swing. She's also going to talk to you about safety a little later.' Without drawing too much attention to Jessie, Tom once again made eye contact and offered Jessie a reassuring smile before continuing. 'Now, I can see some of you have brought golf equipment, does that mean you've played before?' Tom asked. 'Perhaps we could go round and you can all let us know your golf history?'

The empty seats near the door were so close together that sitting down would create a clash of metal so, not wanting to disrupt Tom, Jessie remained standing, half hidden by one of the building's supporting pillars. From this vantage point she could survey the gathered group. Two males and two females sat to the right with faces towards Tom. Three other men sat at a table by the window, all with their faces towards Tom. Two men were leaning against the coffee bar, arms crossed over their chests and staring at the ground. Then, there was a man wearing a large, flat white cap with his arms stretched out on the table in front of him. This man's eyes were focused and fixed on a clean white golf ball which he held in one hand. His hand moved back, and then slowly it released the ball from its grip. His fingers were large, his hand looked strong, the ball, small by comparison, rolled and slowly trickled across the wooden table following a course to his other hand and then, once gathered in, was sent slowly rolling back. Jessie was surprised that someone had brought a golf ball along and the sound of the ball rolling, like a plane flying overhead, thrummed stark and intense in the echoing space. Each time the ball was rolled Tom's voice was ushered into the background. Apart from that, the whole group was hushed and, apart from the golf ball, nothing moved. In fact, Jessie thought, everyone seemed subdued as they took in the instructions and questions from Tom. That was, until Al spoke up:

'I know *all* about bogies!' Al announced in a loud voice. 'Pro's don't like bogies,' he continued, relishing that he knew the term 'bogie' in golf meant that a player had taken one shot too many, but, like a naughty schoolboy, he also knew that bogies, snot or boogars had another meaning, and *that* meaning was likely to make everyone squeal and go, 'Uuurrrgggghhh!' He laughed at his joke and that his knowledge of golf had made it possible to make this play on words.

'Thank you Al,' said Amanda, 'I think we can leave it there.'

Scene 4: Community Sports Centre, 40 minutes later

'What I want you to do,' said Jessie, smiling and then kneeling down in front of Al, 'is to...' Her eyes, now level with Al's knees, brought into vision his thick legs, peachy white skin and the boils like red lumps covering his flesh. From one freshly scratched scab, a small treacly flow of blood was sliding slowly between tangled hairs and other lumps. Jessie thought back to Tom's descriptions of the side effects of antipsychotic medication, she thought about her own puny angst at the side effects of the malaria tablets which had led her question whether trips to Asia were worth it, she wondered how she would feel if her legs looked like that. She wondered whether she should offer a plaster and she hoped Al hadn't seen her notice. These thoughts came and left in the blink of an eye, as she refocused her attention and her eyes on the job at hand and the man in front of her. Looking up at his face, she continued, '... take the club back this far, and follow through to here.' She put her left hand on the floor 10 inches behind the putter head and placed her right hand 15 inches in front on the putter. Then, looking up at Al again, she paused.

Although the room was noisy and there were lots of cheers and balls being dispatched off-course as well as on-course, the groups appeared to be completing their rounds, filling in the score card and, judging by the laughter, enjoying the miss-hits and off-line shots as much as the ones that scored highly. Tom was with the first group, playing the game but also, because he was the organiser and researcher, keeping his radar on continual scan to be attentive to every little blip that might signal a problem. Looking over towards Jessie, he could see her working through the group, reaffirming her earlier coaching points and giving extra input when needed. He could just about hear what she was saying to Al. He was curious, *how* she could be so sure, that if Al took the putter back and through that specific distance it would finish up in the circle. He wondered, mischievously, what would happen if Al swung the club through very quickly and hit the ball really hard, if it would go 100 feet instead of 10 feet. Tom laughed to himself at the prospect of Al's strong arms hitting the ball clean through the back wall. He noticed the way that Jessie worked with Al but continued to made eye contact with the other group members, ensuring they were involved and that they understood the points she was making were applicable to them as well.

'OK, let's see you make that pendulum move again,' she asked. Al responded, moving the club back to the line she had marked and then moved the putter forward to her other hand. 'Excellent!' Jessie encouraged, 'Now I'm going to take my hands away but leave these little marks on the ground for you to follow. Try it again.' Al did as he was told and executed the move perfectly. 'Right,' said Jessie, 'now the final ingredient, see the tempo of my hand as it goes back and through?' Her hand mimicked the rhythm of the putter head, and the speed she wanted Al to follow back and through. 'Can you copy this tempo with the club-head going back and through to those marks?' Al once again complied and executed the task perfectly. 'OK Al, I'm going to ask you to do it again, this time with your eyes closed, and as you do it try to and remember what the move just felt like.' Looking at the group members who were stood behind Al, she then turned her face towards each of them and convincingly reminded them that 'Putting is all about feel,' looking first towards Jeff and then each of the others she said 'Remember, you don't hit the ball, the ball gets in the way of the swing.'

Al closed his eyes as he had been instructed and made the move again, going back and through exactly as Jessie had suggested. 'That's really good,' she said. Tom noticed her tone – she negotiated well the narrow line between encouraging and patronising, he thought. She also sounded like she knew what she was talking about. Of course, she did – not only was Jessie a highly qualified coach but she'd been one of the country's top players and had practised putting for three hours every day for over a decade. Embedded within her body was the exact tempo and distance a putter head should travel. She knew, not because she had read a textbook, but through experience and practice, what the feel of the putter was like, its weight and rhythm, and she wanted Al to succeed in making these distinctions.

'Right, open your eyes and line up the putter head with the target,' she said, 'and then close your eyes again but don't swing till I say.' Al aligned the putter head with the bulls-eye inside the smallest circle 20 feet away, and then closed his eyes. 'Good,' Jessie said, then without Al being aware of it, she placed a golf ball just in front of his putter. The three members of Al's group saw what Jessie had done and in unison tensed and held their breath, mouths open. Was she going to let him hit the ball with his eyes closed? 'OK. Now swing again, Al. Remember that tempo and keep your eyes closed.'

Al swung the putter back and then through but this time, rather than the follow-through moving air, he'd hit something. The feel of the putter making contact with an object and the clunk of metal on plastic astonished Al. Immediately he jumped and opened his eyes. Amazed, he stared in disbelief as his ball rolled gently into the inner circle, gaining him 200 points. Spontaneously he raised his arms in celebration, nearly decapitating Jessie (who was still knelt beside him) with his putter.

'That's my shot!' he shouted out impulsively before turning to the other members of his group, still pointing at his putt. Jessie ducked quickly under the whirling putter before standing up and back, and with a broad smile joined in the applause. 'Two hundred points!' he exclaimed enthusiastically again. He didn't need to tell them. Brian, George and Jeff had witnessed his feat and they too had cheered as the ball entered the inner circle.

From another corner of the room Tom observed the scene. 'Jessie,' he shouted above the bustle, 'have you got a moment?'

Scene 5: a corridor in the sports centre

Paul was outside the putting room, pacing back and forward. Tom saw him leave and popped out to make sure he was alright. Paul had arrived late and had missed the initial talk and instruction.

'Are you getting on alright?' Tom enquired, sitting down on the table outside the room and leaning back against the wall as if he were taking a well-earned rest.

'I just need a cigarette,' Paul responded as he paced quickly back and forth, without making eye contact and drawing quickly and heavily on his cigarette.

'Have you played before?' Tom asked, watching Paul walk to the right and then turn and walk to the left, then turn to the right, then turn to the left. Paul talked very quickly too: 'No, I used to swim. I played football, rugby but never any racket sports, not badminton, tennis or golf.'

'I'll get Jessie to give you a few tips to get you going and you can join my group, we're short of one,' Tom said to Paul at a slower rate, trying to entice him back in to join the group again.

'Alright mate, alright,' Paul said, continuing to talk and walk at a rapid pace, 'I'll be in, in a minute, in a minute.'

After Tom's call, Jessie had crossed the room and stuck her head round the door. She saw Paul pacing. He didn't look over or stop pacing. She glanced over to Tom, who smiled. 'Can you give Paul a little help with his putting when he comes back in?' he asked.

Scene 6: outside Hadden Vale, one hour later

'Are you going to be here next week?' Paul asked Tom.

'Yep, we'll both be here every week.'

'Are you *sure* you're going to be here?' Paul asked again more forcefully.

Tom responded as if he hadn't been asked before, but this time he nodded as well as saying, 'Yep, we'll be taking the session. But we are going to the driving range next week, will you be coming?' Tom asked.

'Alright, mate,' Paul said. 'I'll come.' And then holding out his hand he looked at Tom, 'Nice to meet you, thanks mate.' Paul let go of Tom's hand, turned and left.

Scene 7: café at Hadden Vale, Monday, 3.15 pm

Jeff worked in the café at the day centre. He didn't say much and rarely made eye contact with anyone. But he did his job well enough. When he first came to the centre he wouldn't speak. Now, if someone asks him something he will sometimes respond. Amanda tried drawing him out:

'How's it going, Jeff?' she asked.

'Good thanks,' Jeff said very slowly, very quietly and without looking up.

'Are you going to the golf this week?' she enquired.

'Yes,' he said slowly and without looking up.

'How did you get on last week?'

'Yeah,' he said again slowly, quietly and without looking up, 'good thanks.'

Scene 8: hallway at Hadden Vale, Wednesday 12.30 pm (week 3)

'Everyone's talking about the golf,' Amanda said as Tom and Jessie arrived for the session, 'and two others have signed up this week.' Tom grinned. The first sessions had surpassed his expectations, but this week they were to go to a public driving range and Tom was still working through arrangements in his mind. As he followed Amanda into the day centre he was ticking off items on his mental list. They'd organised a special rate and free refreshments at the range, the minibus could take ten; extras, if there were any, could come with Amanda in her car. Jessie had brought some equipment but the range would supply extra clubs if needed. Tom had enough cash to pay for balls at the range, they would hit shots, then have coffee and cake, they appeared to have everything covered, but still he was a little tense.

They followed Amanda through to the café where the group had assembled prior to departure. Once again Jessie was struck by how still and quiet everyone was.

'OK, time to go,' Amanda announced to the group, 'the mini bus is outside.' She held the door open and one by one the group filed out. Jessie walked along with Paul.

'What's your name again?' he asked.

'Jessie,' she replied with a smile.

'That's a difficult name to remember.' Then Paul asked, 'What's his name?'

'Do you mean Tom?' Jessie replied.

'Yes, Tom, that's it, that's easy, I can remember that.'

'Hi, Al,' Tom said as Al reached the door. 'Have you remembered all those tips you learned last week?' he asked, making conversation.

'Oh yes,' Al replied, 'head still, back and through, pendulum-like.' Tom was impressed.

By the time Al and Tom came to climb into the mini bus the only seats left were up front with the driver.

'Woooh! It's like a school trip!' Tom said, climbing in.

'We were never allowed up front at school,' Al chuckled.

Darren, one of the care co-ordinators, started the engine up. The radio burst into life, interrupting all conversation by blaring out: 'What a *SHHHOT!!!*' It was commentary from Wimbledon. 'She took that at full stretch, a truly *marvellous* passing shot!' the commentator continued. Darren jumped at the unexpected intrusion and tried to turn the volume down but his fumbling only succeeded in retuning the radio. '*SWEEEEET CAROLINE!*' replaced the sport commentary as Neil Diamond's hit blared out from the airwaves. George joined in: 'Bum, bum, bummm! Good times never seem so goooood!' In an instant, the music filled the minibus, transforming the atmosphere. Turning round, his face alight, George began to conduct the others:

'Warm, touchin' warm, reachin' out, touchin' me, touchin' *YOU!*' Encouraged by George, this time, several of the others joined in too:

'Sweeeeet Caroline ... bum bum bummm!'

'That's karaoke music,' Tom whispered to Al. George tilted his head towards Tom:

'Nah! It's a cracker! We used to play this,' he said.

'How d'you mean?' Tom enquired.

'With my band, I used to be in a band,' George continued. 'Yeah, we were wild, I played lead guitar. I always loved this song. But the band didn't!'

'I know the feeling,' Tom laughed, before joining in with the others singing, 'Good times *neevvver* seemed so good.'

The minibus trundled on out of the city, passing warehouses, housing estates, parks, trees, a river, a canal, and onto open roads.

Jessie was at the back squeezed between Jeff and Paul, all three silently gazing at the scenes passing the window, changing from red bricks to open green spaces, their faces flickering as the sunlight darted through the trees, speckling the van and their skin in shade and colour. Their bodies moving as one, as the van rocked and buffeted its inhabitants along the meandering country roads.

'I like to get out,' Paul said to no-one in particular, staring out of the window, his shoulder and body bumping gently against Jessie.

'So do I,' Jessie agreed.

Scene 9: minibus, 10 minutes later

'What do you usually do on Wednesday afternoons?' Jessie asked, interested in the man sat beside her. His thin frame appeared even more frail as it was jolted by the van, and his voice crackled like her great-aunt's as he spoke:

'I usually do my camera course.'

'Oh,' Jessie responded, raising her eyebrows, 'so are you missing that this week?'

'Yes I am,' responded Paul matter-of-factly. 'But I thought the golf would be a good chance to get out. And it's only ten weeks so there's an end in sight and then I will go back to my camera course.'

'Right,' Jessie agreed, slightly confused.

Scene 10: River Park golf range, 15 minutes later

Tom allowed Jessie to take the lead as they entered 'her patch' – the golf range. She jumped out of the van and nodded towards the low-rise building to their left, 'I'll nip in and make sure everything's alright.' The others followed along at a slightly slower pace.

Brian had been hanging back. This was a strange environment. He didn't know what it was going to be like, he didn't know the people at the range, he was being hurried and he didn't like being told what to do. That feeling came again as he climbed out of the van despite trying to focus and going through his strategy on the way. Something dark – a shadow – was following him, creeping closer, it was just behind, he dare not look round. He didn't follow the others in, but walked to the back of the van and lit a cigarette.

'Are you coming, Brian?' Amanda called over, realising Brian was lagging behind.

'I'm just having a cigarette,' he called back, before drawing in a long drag from the roll-up, feeling the effects of the tobacco on his body. It released a little tension. He liked golf, he knew who was teaching, he'd enjoyed it last week, he would hit balls and then they would go back. No problem. Amanda was by his side: 'Oh! It looks really nice, Brian,' she said. Together they walked over to the entrance and through the door. Brian's attention was immediately drawn to the magazine rack.

'Do you know who that is?' he asked, pointing at a magazine. Jessie's eye caught the two coming through the door and Brian pointing at a magazine.

'Who is it?' she called over.

'That's my hero,' Brian said, 'Tiger Woods.'

The driving range owner was golf professional, Ian Stewart. He handed Tom a card for the ball machine with 20 credits and then came out from behind the counter to lead the way. The group followed until a bottleneck, caused by their arrival at the ball machine, halted progress. Ian took a basket and placed it under the mouth of the machine, then he turned to the group, raising his finger and eyebrows.

'It's very important to remember the basket,' he said, before continuing, 'this thing is a bit sticky.' Turning to take the card from Tom and feeding it into the card slot, 'And so ...' he said like a magician, while with a clenched fist making two firm, hard taps on the middle of the ball machine, '... we give it a bit of help!'

Two thumps was all the machine needed to lurch into action. An avalanche of 100 white balls spilled out into the waiting basket – like magic. Ian picked up the now filled basket, gave the card back to Tom and handed the basket to Jessie.

'Voila!' Ian said. 'I'll be in the shop if needed.' Jessie handed the basket to Tom and took the card.

'We'll go down the end,' Jessie said to everyone, but mainly to encourage Tom to lead the way, then turning to Paul who was stood right behind her she took another basket and placed it in position.

'Very important,' she said, 'basket under the hole, card in the slot,' and then with a grin she repeated the instructions: 'And not forgetting two taps here,' she hit the machine twice with her clenched fist and out spewed another 100 balls into the basket. 'OK, your turn,' she said to Paul, passing him the card, 'pass it on when you're finished.' Then she turned and walked off down the range.

Paul took up the challenge as if he'd been given a secret mission with *The A-Team*, and turning round to George, he said, 'Basket under the hole,' and then after putting the basket in place he reiterated the now familiar mantra: 'Card in the slot, and not forgetting two taps here,' he thumped the machine and they all laughed as the balls once again magically appeared like stampeding little sheep into a pen. He then picked up his basket and left George to carry on the game.

Scene 11: on the golf range, 25 minutes later

Tom had a physical education degree, he knew about teaching and he knew how difficult it was to do it well. He observed Jessie as much as he did the group. He didn't expect everyone to stand and give her their complete attention. As he looked around at their eyes, every member of the group was watching intently. They all stood completely still, apart from when she asked them to do warm-up exercises or to make a specific grip. Then, they all joined in and did exactly as she asked. Tom had never had any golf tuition but he'd played with his mates at the pitch 'n' putt years before. Jessie's instructions were clear, they weren't difficult to follow, they might even have seemed a bit obvious. Her group talk was also quite short and she reiterated no more than three points, looking at each member of the group as she spoke.

'So,' Jessie said, coming to the end of her first little group talk, 'always make sure your palm is facing your target, and on the club so that your palm and the club-head are aligning with where you want the ball to go. Place your feet together, like this, and then move the right foot this way, and the left foot this way, to around shoulder width. Then we make the triangle and bend forward like this.' She stood up and smiled at everyone. 'Now, in groups of three, select a bay, remember, take it in turns to hit five shots and help your playing partners if they forget any of the points.' It all sounded quite simple and, as the group dispersed into the driving bays, everyone seemed to know what to do.

Jessie moved into the bay at the end of the range to give George a few pointers. She could see from two bays away that he was struggling and she could see the problem started with his grip. She went down on one knee in front of George and placed her hands on his hands to manoeuvre them into position. She was caught off guard by how thick and puffed up his hands were – no wonder taking a hold was difficult. His hands reminded her of what her rubber gloves looked like when she blew air into them – or perhaps his fingers looked more like Cumberland sausages? The word 'medication' once again flew through her mind. Jessie couldn't help be aware of her own hands, her long slim fingers. Gently moving George's hands she put them in a position where it would be easier to take the club back into position in the back swing. 'How does that feel?' she asked.

'I'd prefer to hold it like this,' George said taking the club in two fists.

'I know,' Jessie said understandingly, 'the problem is though, when you hold it like that, your hands work independently and they don't move into position here, like this.'

She took his hands and arms in hers and moved him halfway through the backswing.

'Ahhh! I see,' he said, taking his eyes off her onto the ground. She took him back to the start position and replaced his hands.

'I know it will feel funny for a while, but keep this feel in your mind and just hit five shots like that to feel and see the difference.' Then turning her head towards the others in the group sharing the bay with George she said, 'Do you see what I'm trying to get George to do? Do you think you can keep checking this as he swings?'

Tom had positioned himself in the next bay and was resting his chin on his arms along the wooden beam that separated the bays. What he saw was like a miracle in George's next shots as they flew beautifully into the air whereas, earlier, they had only been going along the ground and George had been huffing and getting red in the face. But Jessie was already in the next bay working quietly with another player.

Paul came and stood by Tom just in time to see George hit a shot over the 150-yard marker. 'Man that's unbelievable!' he shouted out. 'Great shot mate, that's like the pro's!' It was as though the sun shone from George's face in that moment and his body, it seemed, took a skip.

'OK,' shouted Jessie so everyone could hear, 'we're going to have a little game to finish.' The players all grouped around the end bay and listened as Jessie gave the instructions. They were to take turns in hitting towards different targets to see who could get the closest.

Scene 12: inside the range building, 40 minutes later

The smell hit Ian's nose as he cut open a fresh packet of ground coffee, so he paused a moment to enjoy it. Then he placed three huge spoonfuls of pure Arabica coffee grinds into the cafetière. Leaving it by the kettle, he continued by placing ten cups and saucers on the tray. He opened a drawer and pulled out a paper doily and placed it neatly on the plate before opening a packet of chocolate wheat biscuits which he placed in formation around the plate in spirals. That done, he poured fresh milk into the milk jug and orange juice into the juice jug. Standing back for a moment he surveyed his work and checked that it all looked perfect. Mrs Jenkins came in through the door for her lesson.

'Tim,' Ian said to his assistant, 'make sure you warm the pot before making the tea for Jessie's group. And fill the coffee pot up but leave them to plunge it. I've got to give Mrs Jenkins her lesson now.' With that Ian came out from behind the counter and walked Mrs Jenkins through to the range. Shortly after, Tom came through ahead of the group.

'We're ready for the drinks now,' he said to Tim, who at once reboiled the kettle. As the group came in Tim was handing Tom a complimentary tray of fine coffees, juices and biscuits. Tom put the tray down on a low table surrounded by chairs and then began asking each of the group members what their preference was before handing them a drink.

'Do you want the TV on?' Tim asked, and without waiting for an answer clicked the remote control towards the television and video. The previous year's Open Championship splashed across the screen. Tom was hoping they would all chat, but since some of the group appeared to like it he didn't want to ask to turn it off.

Jessie sat down by George, who was handed a cup of coffee and a biscuit.

'So have you won anything?' George asked, biting into the biscuit.

Tom looked over at Jessie, wondering how she was going to answer. Jessie considered her options. Tom had played down her golf achievements and hadn't advertised them on the promotional literature or talked about them with anyone at the day centre. Jessie was, primarily, a researcher who just happened to be qualified to coach at the highest level in golf. Neither she nor Tom wanted her golf background and notoriety to be a factor in the programme. But judging by the interest George was showing, word had somehow got round and it appeared to her that if she dismissed her golf history it might also seem as if she was dismissing George. So she responded, 'Yes I have.'

'Ooh! What have you won?' George questioned further. Jessie wasn't surprised he was interested, she was used to people asking 'Were you any good?' Then they always asked what she had won. Jessie paused, considering how much to tell – she'd won a lot. Tom looked over, aware of her dilemma and the balance between modesty and boasting. 'Just Google her!' he thought to himself. He contrasted in his mind the high life she had experienced in exotic locations and fancy hotels around the world with the traumatic lives experienced by most members of the group.

'I was European champion twice, English champion, British champion, I won ten tour events and played Solheim Cup,' Jessie said, running through the list without much thought or emotion.

'I hit the pin,' Brian said.

Jessie misheard his remark and replied, 'Yes, I have, one time when it ricocheted into the bunker.'

'Pro's don't like bunkers,' Al chipped in, watching the professional on the TV hit his shot in the bunker, 'cause then they need their sand wedge,' he continued.

'No! *I* hit the pin *today*!' Brian said, making the point that he was talking about his own game, not hers.

'Oh! Sorry, Brian,' Jessie said, feeling embarrassed that she assumed he was asking about her.

'No ...' Brian said.

'I like cheese and ham *sand wedges* though!' Al chipped in again.

'... I hit the 100 yard flag and I hit some shots more than 150,' Brian continued, ignoring the interruptions from Al.

'That's really good,' Jessie said while Al carried on ignoring Brian's contribution to the conversation.

'What's your favourite sand wedge?' Al asked Jessie.

'Ah – tuna and mayo,' Jessie responded amid the crossfire questions.

'No, silly!' Al said laughing and catching her off guard again. 'What type of *sand wedge*,' he said loudly emphasising the words *sand* and *wedge*.

'Oh!' Jessie said laughing, 'I use a Taylor Made sand wedge with 58 degrees loft.'

Brian appeared to be getting bored by the conversation and didn't much like any of the drinks on offer. He wandered over to the counter and asked for a can of coke.

'That's a pound please,' said the assistant.

'A pound!' Brian exclaimed, 'that's very expensive for a can of coke.' His voice boomed across the room and stopped the conversation.

The assistant shrugged. Brian handed over the money and came and sat down.

'That's too expensive,' Brian again said loudly placing the can on the table. 'How can they charge a pound?'

Jessie and Tom exchanged glances. The range had been really good, they'd given them a reduced price on the balls, reserved several bays so the group could be together and provided complimentary coffees, juices and biscuits. Tom felt uneasy with Brian's comment and wanted to quiet him down somehow. Of course, a pound was expensive, especially for someone who had no income.

'I think it's time to go,' Tom announced.

Scene 13: Hadden Vale, Wednesday 11.50 am (week 6)

Darren had been working as a care co-ordinator for thirteen years. At times he was a little worn down by the problems his client group faced. At times, he was a little worn down by the bureaucracy, the tensions between social services and the Trust, and the legal requirements and service guidelines that were forever being rolled in and then rolled out. At times he found some of the clients difficult too and wondered if the money was worth the strain. There was only the smallest window in his tiny office at the top of the building and at this time of year it meant the temperature could be unbearably hot. He looked up at the hands of the clock – again – and continued checking the referral forms, checking the activity groups each individual had signed up for and then cross-referencing the clients' names and attendances each week for every group.

At other times, Darren liked his job. Today, although the morning was tedious he got to play golf all afternoon. This new activity group meant he got to try a game he'd wanted to learn but hadn't had the time or the money to play. With a new baby only ten weeks old he didn't think there would be much time for anything other than helping at home for the next few years. But he also knew there would come a time when he and his son could play golf together, out in the countryside at weekends. Today he was picking up his older daughter Amy from day care after the golf finished. And now he just had to get through these referral forms so he wouldn't need to return to the office after the session. As he worked, he thought about his two kids' future, aware as he looked at the forms how young some of the recent referrals were. He wondered how their parents were coping.

Scene 14: Minibus, 12.55 pm

'Golf's a stupid game!' Al said as his head hit the roof going over the speed bump at the entrance of Hill Park, a local municipal par three course. Darren continued driving a little slower up the long driveway past some of the holes, which were bathed in sunshine and looking very inviting.

'Why d'you say that?' Tom asked. He should have known better. Al was just waiting to bait someone and this time Brian joined in too. 'Because you can't eat your *sand wedges*!' he quipped. Tom smiled, but Al hadn't finished yet. He was sat next to Brian and they began a double act.

'Yes, but that's not all, Brian,' Al continued as if he was giving an interview to the press, 'you can't drink your tee either!'

'And what about your greens?' Brian asked rhetorically before continuing to answer the question himself: 'No, you can't eat your greens 'cause you've got to putt on your greens!'

'Greens you can't eat,' Al exclaimed, 'tees you can't drink and sand wedges you can't eat – how are we going to manage?'

'And without greens, we get no vitamins,' Brian deadpanned back.

'But we have got cake and a flask of coffee!' Tom interrupted, bringing the boys' show to a close.

Jessie was lost in thought, the jokes taking her back to her first golf trip when she was seventeen ... in the back of a Mini Cooper ... the laughter with the other guys, the banter, just like this.

Scene 15: on the course, 25 minutes later

'Being a previous golfer,' Brian exclaimed indignantly, 'I like to hit the ball from where it lies. Texas scramble is not a golf game, I don't like it very much, I want to play my own ball.' Brian stood rooted to his metaphoric spot. He was not going to play Texas scramble, no matter what Jessie said. 'It's not golf!'

Tom was a good negotiator, and so he thought that he would try his diplomacy skills.

'Come on, Brian,' Tom said softly, 'it's just this week to help the others out. Some of the others have never been on a golf course before, it will really help them if they can pick the ball up if they don't hit it very well, and bring it back on the fairway where the better player's shot is and play from there.'

Brian didn't budge, he simply looked away and carried on cleaning his golf ball.

Amanda joined in, 'It's just this week, Brian, next week and all the other weeks you can play your own ball.'

'It's not golf. I know how to play golf and you play the ball from where it lies. That's the game.' He wasn't arguing with them – he wasn't really engaging with them either. He just stated, in matter-of-fact terms, what he was and was not prepared to do.

Scene 16: 10 minutes later

'Am I improving?' Paul asked.

Both Tom and Darren, in unison, exclaimed: 'Yes!'

Tom took the ball away, learning quickly about how to teach golf and what were the critical points for Paul. Then he said, 'Make a shorter, slower swing.' Paul did as he was told. 'Perfect!' Tom said, 'now do the same swing again when I replace the ball.' From 10 feet away, Paul putted with the shorter, slower swing and the ball rolled straight into the hole.

'Yesssss! Great shot!' the group shouted.

In that moment Tom saw the child in Paul. He first tensed then clenched his fists, rising taller by three inches and grinning a huge beam. If that isn't a demonstration of the positive effects of a success experience, Tom thought, nothing is! 'Now how the hell do we get *that* into our research report?' he said to himself.

On the following tee, Paul couldn't seem to get ready to take his shot. He looked serious again, there were no words, he was lost in thought.

'What's up?' Tom asked.

'It's just disbelief,' Paul said, still in a trance, 'that I managed to hole a putt.'

Tom could see that Paul's confidence was low and, although his golf wasn't great, it wasn't terrible. That putt had made a huge difference. Tom had been watching Jessie teach Paul. He noticed, more so than with the others, she spent time trying to get him to use his major muscle groups. Her strategy was obvious to Tom, Paul was so physically fragile that swinging the club seemed really difficult, he had so little strength, even his voice was affected, his wrists couldn't support the club, he had to make use of his shoulders and back. His expectations were about as low as they could be.

Paul tried to tee the ball up but his hand was trembling so much the ball kept falling off. Like Jessie, Tom was well aware of symptoms and medication side effects – muscular hypotension and dyskinesias – but Tom was unsure of whether to take over and tee the ball up for Paul or let him carry on and do it himself. 'I'm bloody useless,' Tom thought to himself, 'they don't teach you how to handle this at uni.'

Scene 17: an hour later

Tom, like many of the others, found his concentration wandering after the first few holes. It was hot, he was mesmerised by the scenery, the quietness and the pleasant pace of play. He had to remind himself to keep offering encouragement and teaching points. But, as the round went on there was little really for him to do as, for the most part, the players he was with clearly knew what they were doing. Part of Tom and Jessie's plan for the golf project was to slowly provide less input in order that, by the time the ten weeks had ended, the group were running things themselves and knew enough about golf, the technique, etiquette and so on, to be able to go off and play independently. So Tom was drawing back a little, but was there to provide an extra hand to those who needed it. Paul found the heat especially difficult so he'd sit down on the grass after each shot and at any other opportunity. Tom helped him gather up his coat, clubs and ball, and there was time just to chat as they walked.

As the afternoon rolled by gently, tired, sweaty bodies lulled off the course towards the wooden benches of the picnic area. Like any other group the golfers all came in with their stories of the day's play.

Jessie was sitting in the picnic area readying drinks and biscuits as, one by one, they slumped down on the wooden benches, dropping golf clubs and superfluous clothing.

'How d'you get on?' Jessie asked, handing a cool drink to Paul.

'That was *way* better than I *ever* thought I would have done!' Paul replied smiling, tipping his head back to down the juice in one go.

'My grip kept going 'cause my hands were sweaty,' interjected Brian as he took the next drink offered by Jessie.

'Aha! You need a glove!' Al suggested, slumping down at the table and waiting to be served.

'My first putt was on line, then it all went pear shaped!' Paul continued, holding out his cup for a refill.

George and Tom were next to arrive. 'I actually hit it today!' George called over as he approached the group, 'I can't believe it!'

Looking down at George's score card, Tom continued the feedback: 'George scored two pars, a couple of fives, the rest fours!' He grinned and passed the score card to Jessie, she handed the cup to George and took the card to give it 'professional' inspection and attention.

'I knew I could do it,' George said, as he accepted a juice from Jessie and lay down on the grassy bank nearby, 'it just takes time to get used to it.' The grass looked too inviting for Paul and Brian so they left the picnic table to Tom and Al and lay down on the grass near George.

Alone now with Al, Tom was aware of an unexpected opportunity. Although uneasy about having to interview these golfers, he was also aware he needed to, ought to...

'Al,' he said, fearful that his question might change the relaxed atmosphere, 'at the beginning we said to everyone that the golf programme is also a research project and we'd like to interview you all about it. Do you ... would you ... be prepared to talk to me ... now ...' he felt himself back-pedalling, 'or some other time?' Al responded immediately, letting Tom off the hook he'd impaled himself on.

'I'll tell you about the golf,' he replied immediately before proceeding to tell more full-throttle stories about the golf that, once again, make Tom laugh. A few moments into one tirade, his voice unexpectedly became quieter and he leaned closer to Tom. 'I know what my legs look like, I can't help that, I know what I look like, I'm not happy about the way I look.' Their intimacy at the table made Tom feel awkward. Should he touch Al? Make contact? Try to make him feel that he wasn't 'unclean'? That his legs weren't so bad. What he wanted to do was to reach out in some way, to do or say something, but the words he thought of seemed useless and pathetic.

'I can't handle people being mocking, mocking me.' Al continued to talk while scratching the sores on his lower legs which were now bleeding again. 'I worry over my appearance. I often feel anxious, get nervous with groups.'

In these few moments Tom had seen Al turn from a witty comedian to a serious, contemplative thinker. He'd heard him make observations that the smartest ethnographer might miss. He'd seen Al open a window to his vulnerabilities. Although wary of where his questions might lead, Tom now felt compelled walk on with Al, to at least provide an opportunity for him to speak further, if he wanted. 'So have you,' Tom hesitated, he'd seen so many good things happen in the previous weeks, but their closeness and this moment compelled him to dig beneath the happy surface, 'have you felt like that with the golf group?'

Al didn't tiptoe in the moral quagmire that was threatening to suffocate Tom. 'Yes,' he replied, 'sometimes. In the golf sessions, unfamiliar people, you know, that troubles me.' Al raised his voice a little again and leaned back away from Tom. 'I like it lighthearted. I can't stand intensity.' Tom nodded, and continued to carefully focus his dark eyes fully on Al. 'I didn't like that game last week,' Al continued, 'nearest the pin. I don't like competition, who's winning, who's losing. I've never been used to intensity.'

Scene 18: 15 minutes later

Sat on the grass, most of the group seemed tired and relaxed, except for Darren.

'Come on everyone!' he said, looking once again at his watch, trying to chivvy them along. They were past the scheduled finish time and Darren could already visualise his three-year-old daughter crying, left on her own at childcare because daddy failed to pick her up on time. A great carer I am, he thought to himself.

There was a queue to get out onto the main road. The difficulty getting out in the traffic made Darren even more aware that he was late. His shoulders and neck tightened with each passing second, increasing his silent fury; over and over in his head he wondered why he'd let the situation get so unruly, time-wise. Looking once more at the traffic he considered his options: return the way they had come or squeeze over the pavement past the queuing cars. Knowing the locality well, he took a chance on returning via the Great Hampton Bridge which, because they were going against the traffic, surely wouldn't be busy. The bus creaked and groaned as it was levered around amidst the inching vehicles, causing the occupants to be thrown from side to side by the overzealous suspension. The barrage of beeping horns from annoyed car drivers made everyone aware this manoeuvre wasn't planned but, at last, the breeze funnelled in through the open windows as they headed at speed along the empty road leading to the bridge.

The conversation had dried up with the commotion of the traffic, as the group sensed Darren's mood had changed: his eyebrows furrowed, his grip on the wheel making his veins bulge, the gear leaver rammed into place at each gear change. But, like children watching their parents argue, there was little Tom or Jessie could do about the situation. They sat quietly, trying to look like they weren't observing these changes, but they monitored every breath. Neither of them could really hear what was being said at the back of the bus, and at first it seemed just like a quiet unimportant conversation.

Then Paul shouted forward: 'I can't go over the bridge!' He spoke very quickly and was clinging to his coat. He spoke these words only once more but the reaction of those around him brought a gravity to the situation which Tom and Jessie hadn't seen before. They glanced towards each other and then towards the back of the van and then towards the front.

Amanda leaned over and said something quietly to Darren, who said something quietly back. Neither Tom nor Jessie could make out what was said. They glanced at each other again, frozen out of the loop. George called from the back, 'Paul can't go over the bridge!' Jessie and Tom looked back.

Darren sat hardened at the wheel, continuing to drive. Paul sat wide-eyed and rigid in the back, unable to go over the bridge. 'It'll be OK, Paul,' George said soothingly, as they drove across the bridge.

Scene 19: café at Hadden Vale, Monday, 11.00 am

'How are you doing, Jeff?' Amanda asked as she picked up a mug of tea from the café.
  'Good thanks,' Jeff replied without looking up.
  'How was golf last week?' Amanda continued, trying to maintain a conversation.
  'Good thanks,' Jeff quietly replied.
  'Are you coming again tomorrow?'
  'Yes.'
Brian walked into the café and, as he did so, Jeff looked up, a huge smile creeping across his face. Jeff shouted out in a high-pitched voice, 'You're *the pro* who hit the ball two hundred yards at the range!' He pointed over towards Brian, still smiling, as he exclaimed, '*And* you holed that huge putt last week!' Then he stood there for a moment, holding his smile.
  'Yes! I am *the white tiger*!' Brian laughed in response. The two men smiled at each other, holding their gaze for a moment, before Jeff's eyes returned to the counter and he went on with his work in silence.

Scene 20: café at Hadden Vale, Wednesday 12.35 pm (week 9)

'I've got photos!' George shouted as he entered the café waving an oblong envelope.
'Oooh, let's see!' Jessie said, looking over. The group bunched together, bringing seats and bodies closer.
  'Any of me there?' asked Brian leaning his head over the envelope like a cook over a boiling pot.
  'Yeah, yeah, we got everyone!' George said. 'Tom and Jessie, Amanda and Darren too.' The first photo was of Jessie and George, stood together. He was smiling, holding a golf club, she had her funny little sunhat on, was wearing shorts and a sun top and, she thought, her legs looked really tanned. It was the sort of photo that had been taken of her a million times in pro-am and golf events, there was nothing special about this one, except there was everything special about it. Unlike her other golf photos, she could never use this one: he was a participant, she was a researcher, he was supposed to be anonymous. Reluctantly she passed the photo on before taking the next one from George.
  'Hey, look at this one!' Jessie exclaimed, her thoughts now on Brian on the tee.
  'You got me in full swing!' Brian took Jessie's hand and pulled it round to get a better view.
  'Great swing, Brian!' she said. 'You look like a pro!'
  'Yes,' he said, with an air of superiority, 'you're not the first to comment on my swing.' Brian took the photo and passed it on.

'Aha, I see what you mean, a real pro,' said Al, taking the photograph.

'Oh no! I remember that hole, it was a killer!' Brian said as the next photo was passed along. 'Who's that there, George?'

Peering over, George looked at the person Al's finger was pointing at, 'Um, it looks like Paul. He stopped coming, he didn't like going over the bridge.'

'Shame,' Al continued, looking at the photo, ''cause from the photo it looks like he's holed a huge putt, look at the grin on his face!'

Jessie took the photo, she remembered Paul, his huge smile and arms aloft captured in the photo. She wondered what he was doing now, she wondered if she should have done more to get him back playing golf after the bridge episode. Or should she have done more to make Darren go another way? Or was it just one of those things?

'What about this one, lads?' said George, passing another photo round. There was a burst of simultaneous laughter.

'I remember that!' Al said to Brian, 'You look like that American golfer.'

'Tiger Woods?' Brian asked.

'Yeah, yeah, Tiger Woods!' Al agreed.

'I *am* the Tiger!' Brian continued, 'Even on the greens!' They all laughed again as Brian drew attention to how his long hitting on the fairway was not a blessing on the greens and usually made the ball fly *past* the hole rather than into it.

George handed the photo on. 'Ooooh dear, you're not gonna like this one, Brian,' George said looking closely at the next photo.

'Photos don't do us any favours do they?' said Brian, looking at the photo Jessie was holding. She passed it on. The group became quiet.

'I've got to lose some weight,' Brian said, breaking the silence, and then, 'I've got to come off medication.'

Scanning the photo Al joined in, 'Same here.'

'I stopped taking mine,' said George, 'I got a stash like, for emergencies,' he continued, looking at the photos still in his hand.

'Yeah, me too, just for emergencies like.'

To Jessie it sounded like they all had a stash of medication for emergencies. It also felt like a window to their experience had been opened to her as she sat there listening to them all discuss their bodies, appearances, medication and self-management. She wondered how she would feel; she wondered if it was safe to be giving up medication or keeping 'stashes'. As a researcher, this moment was a real nugget, she was excited with her find and couldn't wait to tell Tom. But like catching a glimpse of a parent with no clothes on, she was also uneasy at what she had seen – that these men had exposed themselves to her, metaphorically naked, open and trusting. Would sharing this story be breaking their trust? There was no resolution.

Concluding thoughts

A question some readers might be asking at this point is: What does this story tell us about the practice and provision of physical activity and sport for mental health? It would be futile for us to offer a 'summary' of the insights the story provides – this would negate our rationale for using a storied approach which is rooted in the conviction that certain kinds of understandings are best expressed through a story form. For us, particular truths and knowledge are expressed within each scene and, to appreciate these, it is necessary for the reader to 'think with' – rather than analyse – those scenes. Lori Neilsen (2008, p. 96) expresses well what a reader might 'take from' an effective arts-informed representation:

> A reader does not take away three key points or five examples. A reader comes away with the resonance of another's world, in the way we emerge from the reading of a poem or a novel, from a film screening or a musical event – physically transported or moved, often unaware of the architecture or structure that created the experience, our senses stimulated, our spirit and emotion affected.

We hope that you find our story to be effective in this regard and that, as Frank (2000b) suggests, it might have provided a picture of things that allows you to see everything else differently. If this process 'works', Frank explains, 'the picture itself does not convince us; rather it destabilizes our old ways of seeing and thus allows new images into our awareness' (p. 149).

For us, this story comes closest to preserving two particular qualities which we have appreciated through conducting this research. First, the story provides a heightened awareness of an intricate web of *connections* – between people, places, experiences, events, objects and biographies – which are central to the relationship between sport/physical activity and mental health. The procedures of traditional scientific forms of measurement and analysis tend to focus narrowly on phenomena and events which have been removed from their everyday context. As a result, connected elements can come to appear disparate and unconnected. In contrast, using a story form to represent observations and experiences in situ helps to *reveal* and *restore* important connections – both for the writer (through the writing process) and, hopefully, for the reader (through the finished text).

Second, the story form allows the preservation of a degree of *openness* which stands in contrast to more traditional forms of scientific writing where interpretations and conclusions tend to be tightly defined and 'finalised' (Sparkes, 2002). In our story, the quality of openness is faithful to our experiences of practice and provision: time and again, chance or unpredictable happenings seemed to hold importance for individuals within the group. Although the meaning and significance of these events is difficult or impossible to pin down, this does not imply that they were unimportant.

For example, it is somewhat ironic that although, as researchers, Tom and Jessie were monitoring the participants, the participants were also (through taking photographs) monitoring the researchers and each other. While these photographs could not be published for ethical reasons, the final episode of the story portrays something important taking place through sharing and talking about the photographs. The photographs seemed to act as a catalyst for participants to reflect on (among other things) their bodies, their medication regimes and 'stashes'. While we recognise that *something* important is happening at this moment, it is impossible for us as researchers to *specify* the meaning of these events for the individuals concerned. The story form allows these kinds of event to be included in order that readers might form their own interpretations in the light of their own experience.

Some mental health literature suggests that a degree of openness is important when it comes to recovery (e.g. Anthony, 1993; Deegan, 1996). Chadwick (2009, p. 126), for example, observes how 'In the sinister multi-faceted diamond that is schizophrenic psychosis, one simply does *not* know, in the foresight situation, whatever meta-analyses and randomised controlled trials may state, which avenues a particular person will find productive.' From this perspective, a failure to remain open threatens to close down possibilities that particular individuals might find important in their recovery through *finalising* people's lives. While it is not the case that the story has nothing to say regarding the contribution of sport to the lives of people with mental health difficulties (for us, some of our most important insights are couched within particular scenes), neither can the story be seen as a finalised account which *states as fact* the nature of the physical activity–mental health relationship. Monologues of this kind threaten dialogical conversation and reflection because they exclude alternatives through promoting a singular, finalised representation of reality. On this basis, 'the research report must always understand itself not as a final statement of who the research participants are, but as one move in a continuing dialogue through which those participants will continue to form themselves, as they continue to become who they may yet be' (Frank, 2005, pp. 966–7). We hope this chapter provides a useful example of this work.

Looking to the future

12

From the outset, we had two broad aims for this book. The first was to shed some light on the processes by which physical activity and sport can contribute to recovery in the context of mental health problems. As we discussed in chapter 1, 'survivor' accounts suggest that several themes characterise the recovery process. These focus on the need to: (i) rebuild social roles and relationships; (ii) develop meaning and purpose in one's life; (iii) recreate a positive sense of self and identity; (iv) change one's attitudes, values and goals; (v) enact, acquire and demonstrate ability; (vi) pursue personal interests, hopes and aspirations; and (vii) develop and maintain a sense of hopefulness about one's future. Throughout the book we have provided illustrations of how – for different people, at different times, in differing contexts – involvement in physical activity or sport can contribute to meeting some (or even all) of these diverse recovery needs.

We have described three distinct ways through which physical activity or sport can contribute to recovery:

- For those individuals who previously held (or currently hold) an athletic identity, re-engaging in physical activity or sport can facilitate the reconstruction of a valued sense of self or identity that has been lost or damaged through the experience of mental illness.
- For others who perhaps do not hold an athletic identity, 'adventure' experiences through physical activity or sport can stimulate the creation and sharing of new life stories around the experience of action, achievement and relationships.
- For others, physical activity or sport can serve as a vehicle or stepping stone for particular outcomes (e.g. improved fitness, weight loss, social connectedness) which help individuals to – in one way or another – move on in life.

Our work has led us to the conclusion that the ways in which physical activity and sport contribute to recovery is closely related to the meaning that the activity holds for the individual concerned. To provide personally meaningful – and hence beneficial – opportunities it is therefore necessary to pay close attention to the history, needs, preferences and aspirations of each individual. It is simply not the case that a standardised 'prescription' of exercise will be beneficial to all people, or even all people with a particular diagnosis. Rather, we now understand, the ways in which physical activity or sport contributes to recovery are varied, complex and person-specific. So too are the recovery needs of people with a mental illness. On this basis, we suggest that the potential of physical activity and sport to contribute to recovery is *dependent* upon the point that participation means different things to different people. Put another way, the variation and uniqueness inherent in the physical activity–mental health relationship is critical to its success – precisely because it allows individuals to experience the kinds of benefits that match their own recovery needs.

Our second aim for the book was to generate some insights regarding how physical activity and sport provision might be made in ways that are most likely to be experienced as beneficial. In chapter 7 we described some features of the culture of sport and physical activity which, on the basis of our own research (Douglas & Carless, 2006, 2009a; Carless & Douglas, 2009a), are more likely to *cause* mental health difficulties than help with them. In particular, an orientation towards performance outcomes can be harmful. In its place we have illustrated throughout the book how, in order to be beneficial, the ethos, climate, coaching and leadership of physical activity and sport initiatives is better oriented towards action, achievement, discovery and/or relationships. Through presenting, in Part III, practitioner interviews and a fictionalised story we hope to have revealed some of the subtleties and complexities of effective provision in a way that provides some direction and ideas for professionals in mental health and sport and exercise.

Developing research

How then, we ask ourselves, should we – together – be taking this field of research forward? Do we need scientific 'proof' of the benefits of physical activity for people with mental health problems? Should we invest in clinical trials which explore which activities produce what types of benefit? Should we implement interventions to explore the most effective 'prescription' of exercise in terms of frequency, intensity and duration? Should we fund epidemiological studies which count how many people experience symptom relief and how many do not? Or should research focus on the cost-effectiveness of activity in comparison to other forms of 'treatment'? In light of the research we have presented in the previous chapters, we know exercise is valued and valuable in the lives of some people who have mental health problems. We also know that the type of activity that 'works' depends on the individual – their physical activity history, lifestyle, preferences, aspirations, social networks and local opportunity. On the basis of our work in this field to date, we believe that there are several pressing questions which future research in this field could beneficially focus upon. These include:

- *How can physical activity and sport opportunities be tailored to be more appealing to those people who are currently inactive?* Women and ethnic minority groups have been reported to have low levels of engagement with physical activity and/or mental health services and little physical activity–mental health research has been conducted with these groups. How might sport and activity provision be presented, promoted and managed in order to be more appealing, interesting and rewarding for these persons? Consideration might be given to both the *forms* of activity/sport which are offered and the *ways in which* provision is made and sessions are run.

- *How might the balance between support and independence be negotiated?* While there are moves towards increasing social inclusion through community-based sport and exercise participation, we are at the same time concerned that provision in sport and leisure centres may be too advanced for those who are most unwell.

- *How might we better manage transition and progression so that valued social and support networks are not lost when a person is discharged?* Several participants in our research have experienced difficulties on discharge because they are no longer able to access physical activity and sport run by mental health services. At this difficult time, these individuals describe losing the very activity and social network that has helped them recover. What ongoing opportunities could be set up? How might sport enthusiasts be supported in maintaining an ongoing role through becoming (for example) coaches or mentors?

- *In what ways can the quality of coaching provision in mental health contexts be improved and/or extended?* One approach might be through more extensive coach education regarding mental health, cultural issues in sport and exercise, and concepts such as diversity, equity and inclusion.

- *How might stigma in society regarding mental illness be challenged in order to improve the community-based sport/activity experiences of people with mental health problems?* Possible approaches might include coach/peer advocacy, education and awareness raising, circulation of alternative stories of sport/exercise and mental health.

- *What can we learn from the voices of individuals who access sport and physical activity from within mental health services?* What might we learn from those who are resistant to sport and physical activity?

- *How might other forms of physical activity (e.g. dance or outdoor activity) contribute to recovery?* To date, most research has focused on common forms of exercise (e.g. walking, gym, running) and sport (e.g. football, golf). Alternative cooperative activities offer a different emphasis to more competitively oriented activities which may be appealing to some people who are currently disinclined towards activity.

It has become clear to us through the varied analytical and representational approaches we have employed in our research and through the chapters of this book that, as Richardson (2000) and Eisner (2008) suggest, the *ways* in which we gather, analyse and represent our research 'data' shapes the *kinds* of knowledge we construct through our work. In other words, the way we *do* research shapes the 'findings' we produce. This interplay has significant long-term consequences in terms of both the processes and products of human and social science research. In relation to this point, Chadwick (2009, p. 130) writes 'Materialistic science and atheism compel and challenge investigators to explore that in people which is most animal and machine-like. Art, however, compels and challenges us to seek that which is most human.' On this basis, we suggest that research which draws on artistic values and approaches (such as ethnodrama, ethnographic fiction, autoethnography, songwriting and poetic representation) is a necessary component of future research if constructive, balanced, ethical, humane and inclusive research is to be conducted and disseminated.

Developing practice and provision

At this point in time we see two priority areas in terms of developing the practice and provision of sport and physical activity in mental health contexts. The first of these concerns what appears to be a tension between current moves towards independence and community-based provision and some individuals' need for specialist provision and/or support. While, on the one hand, community integration is a positive move because it can lead to sustainable participation which is rooted within one's locality, on the other hand it risks leaving individuals without specialist support in an activity session which may be beyond their current abilities. We have seen how 'stepping stone' groups have an important role to play in this regard because they initiate social networks within a protected physical activity space. This can lead to several possible benefits, not least a feeling of shared experience and common ground. In the following excerpt, one individual (who attended a recent evaluation focus group) describes the difference between an activity group in a mental health setting and voluntary work in the community:

> Sometimes when I self-harm, I feel less judged on my bruises or marks at the group than I do with other people. When I go to my volunteering at the charity shop, I wear long sleeves to cover my arms, whereas at badminton I feel comfortable wearing a t-shirt. I think if we talked too much about our illness/problems to so-called 'normal people' they might think we are a bit self-obsessed. Whereas in the group, because we all have similar problems, it is good to share it with each other.

We are aware that attending a group with people from similar backgrounds may bring both benefits and problems. However, as the excerpt above suggests, shared experience can mean an individual doesn't feel the need to 'cover up' in the way they might in other groups. Knowing that one's needs (e.g. needing 'time out' on days when one is feeling more unwell) will be recognised and respected leads people to feel more confident attending an activity group on 'bad days' as well as 'good days'. Ideally, this kind of recognition and individual focus would be present in *any* activity group in a community or mental health setting. Our concern is whether there is yet sufficient awareness among community-based sport/activity leaders, instructors and coaches of these kinds of issues. At some time in the future our society may become sufficiently informed and accepting to negate this concern. In the meantime, we suggest that it is important not to move too quickly, that people who are using mental health services (or have recently been discharged) continue to be offered safe and supportive 'stepping stone' activity environments which are cognisant of the kinds of difficulties their mental health problems may raise.

The second priority area, as we see it, concerns the availability and provision of educational opportunities for coaches and activity leaders who work in mental health settings. The qualities and skills of the coach or activity leader are likely to be crucial in terms of the effectiveness of any activity. The activity leader or coach has the opportunity to integrate potentially disparate individuals into a functioning group, educate group members and support and encourage those who may be unsure about their involvement. At present, however, the majority of training programmes for coaches seem to focus primarily on performance outcomes (e.g. development that leads towards the elite or professional level). What is needed instead, we suggest, are educational opportunities which will help coaches and leaders develop skills and strategies to meet the needs of groups who have been previously marginalised or excluded from sport and physical activity.

We suggest a broad shift in the ethos and goals of coach education opportunities is needed to move away from the values of a performance narrative (e.g. competition, winning, sacrifice, performance outcomes) towards an alternative set of values related to meeting individual needs through action, achievement, discovery and relationships. Education of this kind will require coaches and leaders to explore sport and activity in an open-minded way – a type of learning that is facilitated by an environment where one is allowed (and even encouraged) to be creative, to imagine off-the-wall approaches and to take chances. Educational initiatives of this kind have the potential to facilitate problem-based learning and reflective practice that can lead to professional development and improved practice (see Douglas & Carless, 2008a, 2009b). It is beholden on sport governing bodies to ensure that incentives are put in place so coaches and activity specialists who seek to support these widening participation goals do not lose out on either career progression or remuneration.

A closing thought

Having purposes and goals for our physical activity and sport participation (be they improved mental health, weight loss, social connectedness, improved fitness, better performance) is all well and good – this approach has its place. Yes, it is important to be active to maintain health. Yes, many sportspeople gain satisfaction from improving their performance. Yes, social inclusion does (of course) matter. It sometimes appears, however, that as a consequence of the contemporary quest for 'evidence of effectiveness', the purposes, outcomes and goals of participation come to be seen as more important than the *process* of being involved. We worry that the current climate requires those running sessions to make claims for what physical activity and sport can bring and then invest a great deal of energy and time in evaluating the programme according to these outcomes. It is important, we think, to remember that sport and physical activity are also *games*. Oftentimes, involvement is most beneficial to the human spirit when it is *ludic*: it perhaps requires no further outcome other than that it is fun and enjoyable in the moment, that it makes us laugh like a child, that it surprises and entertains. If we try to pin down and control activities too much, we threaten the potentially essential elements of enjoyment, connection, surprise, inspiration, creativity and spontaneity.

References

Allison, D.B., Mentore, J.L., Heo, M., Chandler, L., Cappelleri, J.C., Infante, M.C., & Weiden, P.J. (1999). Antipsychotic-induced weight gain: A comprehensive research synthesis. *American Journal of Psychiatry*, **156**, 1686–1696.

Angrosino, M. (1998). *Opportunity House: Ethnographic Stories of Mental Retardation*. Walnut Creek, CA: Alta Mira.

Anthony, W. (1993). Recovery from mental illness. *Innovations and Research*, **2**(3), 17–25.

Apitzsch, E. (1998). Gender and sports participation. In R. Seiler & E. Apitzsch (Eds.), FEPSAC Monograph Series #2. ISSN 1562–1278.

Bakan, D. (1966). *The Duality of Human Existence*. Chicago, IL: Rand McNally.

Baker-Brown, S. (2006). A patient's journey: Living with paranoid schizophrenia. *BMJ*, **333**, 636–638.

Baldwin, C. (2005). Narrative, ethics and people with severe mental illness. *Australian and New Zealand Journal of Psychiatry*, **39**, 1022–1029.

Bedi, R.P. (1999). Depression: An inability to adapt to one's perceived life distress? *Journal of Affective Disorders*, **54**(1–2), 225–234.

Beebe, L.H., Tian, L., Morris, N., Goodwin, N., Allen, S.S., & Kuldau, J. (2005). Effects of exercise on mental and physical health parameters of persons with schizophrenia. *Issues in Mental Health Nursing*, **26**, 661–676.

Behar, R. (1993). *Translated Woman: Crossing The Border With Esperanza's Story*. Boston: Beacon.

Biddle, S.J.H., Fox, K.R., & Boutcher, S.H. (Eds.) (2000). *Physical Activity and Psychological Well-being*. London: Routledge.

Blinde, E., & Stratta, T. (1992). The 'sport career death' of college athletes: Involuntary and unanticipated sport exits. *Journal of Sport Behavior*, **15**, 3–20.

Blinde, E., Taub, D., & Han, L. (1994). Sport as a site for women's group and societal empowerment: Perspectives from the college athlete. *Sociology of Sport Journal*, **11**, 51–59.

Bochner, A. (1997). It's about time: Narrative and the divided self. *Qualitative Inquiry*, **3**(4), 418–438.

Brewer, B., Van Raalte, J., & Linder, D. (1993). Athletic identity: Hercules' muscle or Achilles heel? *International Journal of Sport Psychology*, **24**, 237–254.

Brooks, P. (1994). *Psychoanalysis and Storytelling*. Oxford: Blackwell.

Bruner J.S. (1986). *Actual Minds, Possible Worlds*. Cambridge. MA: Harvard University Press.

Bryson, L. (1987). Sport and the maintenance of masculine hegemony. *Women's Studies International Forum*, **10**(4), 349–360.

Callaghan, P. (2004). Exercise: A neglected intervention in mental health care? *Journal of Psychiatric and Mental Health Nursing*, **11**, 476–483.

Cantor, W., & Bernay, T. (1992). *Women in Power: The Secrets of Leadership*. Boston, MA: Houghton Mifflin.

Carless, D. (2003). *Mental Health and Physical Activity in Recovery*. Doctoral dissertation, University of Bristol.

Carless, D. (2007). Phases in physical activity initiation and maintenance among men with serious mental illness. *International Journal of Mental Health Promotion*, **9**(2), 17–27.

Carless, D. (2008). Narrative, identity, and recovery from serious mental illness: A life history of a runner. *Qualitative Research in Psychology*, **5**(4), 233–248.

Carless, D. (in press). Who the hell was *that*? Stories, bodies and actions in the world. *Qualitative Research in Psychology*.

Carless, D., & Douglas, K. (2004). A golf programme for people with severe and enduring mental health problems. *Journal of Mental Health Promotion*, **3**(4), 26–39.

Carless, D., & Douglas, K. (2008a). Narrative, identity and mental health: How men with serious mental illness re-story their lives through sport and exercise. *Psychology of Sport and Exercise*, **9**(5), 576–594.

Carless, D., & Douglas, K. (2008b). The role of sport and exercise in recovery from mental illness: Two case studies. *International Journal of Men's Health*, **7**(2), 137–156.

Carless, D., & Douglas, K. (2008c). Social support for and through exercise and sport in a sample of men with serious mental illness. *Issues in Mental Health Nursing*, **29**, 1179–1199.

Carless, D., & Douglas, K. (2008d). The contribution of exercise and sport to mental health promotion in serious mental illness: An interpretive project. *International Journal of Mental Health Promotion*, **10**(4), 5–12.

Carless, D., & Douglas, K. (2009a). 'We haven't got a seat on the bus for you' or 'All the seats are mine': Narratives and career transition in professional golf. *Qualitative Research in Sport and Exercise*, **1**(1), 51–66.

Carless, D., & Douglas, K. (2009b). Stepping out of the box: How stories can inspire growth, development, and change. *Annual Review of High Performance Coaching and Consulting* **2009**, 175–185.

Carless, D., & Douglas, K. (2009c). Opening doors: Poetic representation of the sport experiences of men with severe mental health difficulties. *Qualitative Inquiry*, **15**(10), 1547–1551.

Carless, D., & Faulkner, G. (2003). Physical activity and mental health. In J. McKenna & C. Riddoch (Eds.), *Perspectives on Health and Exercise* (pp. 61–82). Houndsmills: Palgrave Macmillan.

Carless, D., & Sparkes, A. (2008). The physical activity experiences of men with serious mental illness: Three short stories. *Psychology of Sport and Exercise*, **9**(2), 191–210.

Carter-Morris, P., & Faulkner, G. (2003). A football project for service users: The role of football in reducing social exclusion. *Journal of Mental Health Promotion*, **2**, 24–31.

Chadwick, P.K. (1997a). *Schizophrenia: The Positive Perspective*. London: Routledge.

Chadwick, P.K. (1997b). Recovery from psychosis: Learning more from patients. *Journal of Mental Health*, **6**, 577–588.

Chadwick, P.K. (2001a). Psychotic consciousness. *International Journal of Social Psychiatry*, **47**(1), 52–62.

Chadwick, P.K. (2001b). *Personality as Art: Artistic Approaches in Psychology*. Ross-on-Wye, UK: PCCS Books.

Chadwick, P.K. (2006). Wilde's creative strategies. *The Wildean*, **29**, 28–39.

Chadwick, P.K. (2007). Freud meets Wilde: A playlet. *The Wildean*, **31**, 2–22.

Chadwick, P.K. (2009). *Schizophrenia: The Positive Perspective (second edition)*. London: Routledge.

Charon, R. (2006). The self-telling body. *Narrative Inquiry*, **16**(1), 191–200.

Charmaz, K. (1991). *Good Days, Bad Days: The Self in Chronic Illness and Time*. New Brunswick, NJ: Rutgers University Press.

Clandinin, D.J. & Murphy, M.S. (2007). Looking ahead: Conversations with Elliot Mishler, Don Polkinghorne, and Amia Lieblich. In D.J. Clandinin (Ed.), *Handbook of Narrative Inquiry* (pp. 632–650). Thousand Oaks, CA: Sage.

Coleman, R. (1999). *Recovery: An Alien Concept*. Gloucester, UK: Handsell Publishing.

Conner, M., & Armitage, C. (2000). *The Social Psychology of Food*. Buckingham, UK: Open University Press.

Corrigan, P., & Phelan, S. (2004). Social support and recovery in people with serious mental illness. *Community Mental Health Journal*, **40**(6), 513–523.

Crone, D. (2007). Walking back to health: A qualitative investigation into service users' experiences of a walking project. *Issues in Mental Health Nursing*, **28**, 167–183.

Crone, D., & Guy, H. (2008). 'I know it's only exercise, but to me it is something that keeps me going': A qualitative approach to understanding mental health service users' experiences of sports therapy. *International Journal of Mental Health Nursing*, **17**, 197–207.

Crone, D., Heaney, L., Herbert, R., Morgan, J., Johnston, L., & Macpherson, R. (2004). A comparison of lifestyle behaviour and health perceptions of people with severe mental illness and the general population. *Journal of Mental Health Promotion*, **3**(4), 19–25.

Crone, D., Smith, A., & Gough, B. (2005). 'I feel totally at one, totally alive and totally happy': A psycho-social explanation of the physical activity and mental health relationship. *Health Education Research*, **20**(5), 600–611.

Crossley, M. (2000). *Introducing Narrative Psychology: Self, Trauma and the Construction of Meaning*. Maidenhead, UK: Open University Press.

Dant, T. (2001). Fruitbox/toolbox: Biography and objects. *Auto/Biography*, **IX**, 1 & 2, 11–20.

David Lloyd Leisure. (2009). http://www.davidlloyd.co.uk/home/activities/classes/conditioning,12/08/2009

Davidson, L. (2003). *Living Outside Mental Illness*. New York: New York University Press.

Davidson, L., O'Connell, M., Tondora, J., Lawless, M., & Evans, A. (2005). Recovery in serious mental illness: A new wine or just a new bottle? *Professional Psychology: Research and Practice*, **36**(5), 480–487.

Davidson, L., & Roe, D. (2007). Recovery from versus recovery in serious mental illness: One strategy for lessening confusion plaguing recovery. *Journal of Mental Health*, **16**(4), 459–470.

Davies, B. (2001). Becoming male or female. In S. Jackson & S. Scott (Eds.), *Gender* (pp. 280–290). London: Routledge.

De Botton, A. (2000). *The Consolations of Philosophy*. London: Hamish Hamilton.

Deegan, P. (1996). Recovery as a journey of the heart. *Psychiatric Rehabilitation Journal*, **19**(3), 91–97.

Deegan, P. (1997). Recovery and empowerment for people with psychiatric disabilities. *Social Work in Health Care*, **25**(3), 11–24.

Denzin, N.K. (2003). *Performance Ethnography*. Thousand Oaks, CA: Sage.

Department for Culture, Media and Sport (2002). *Game Plan: A strategy for delivering Government's sport and physical activity objectives*. London: Strategy Unit. Crown Copyright.

Department for Culture, Media and Sport (2008). *Playing to Win: A New Era for Sport*. London: HMSO. Crown Copyright.

Department of Health (2003). *Promoting Mental Health: Strategy and Action Plan 2003–2008*. Belfast: Department of Health, Social Services and Public Safety. Crown Copyright.

Department of Health (2004). *At Least Five a Week: A Report from the Chief Medical Officer*. London: HMSO. Crown Copyright.

Department of Health. (2009). *A Systematic Review of the Evidence Base for Developing a Physical Activity and Health Legacy from the London 2012 Olympic and Paralympic Games*. London: HMSO. Crown Copyright.

Douglas, K. (2004). *What's the Drive in Golf? Motivation and Persistence in Professional Tournament Golfers*. Doctoral dissertation, University of Bristol.

Douglas, K. (2009). Storying my self: Negotiating a relational identity in professional sport. *Qualitative Research in Sport and Exercise*, **1**(2), 176–190.

Douglas, K., & Carless, D. (2005). *Across the Tamar: Stories from Women in Cornwall*. (CD) Bristol, UK: Self-produced.

Douglas, K., & Carless, D. (2006). Performance, discovery, and relational narratives among women professional tournament golfers. *Women in Sport and Physical Activity Journal*, **15**(2), 14–27.

Douglas, K., & Carless, D. (2008a). Using stories in coach education. *International Journal of Sports Science and Coaching*, **3**(1), 33–49.

Douglas, K., & Carless, D. (2008b). Nurturing a performative self. *Forum Qualitative Sozialforschung/Forum: Qualitative Social Research*, **9**(2), Art. 23, http://www.qualitative-research.net/fqs-texte/2–08/08–2-23-e.htm

Douglas, K., & Carless, D. (2008c). The team are off: Getting inside women's experiences in professional sport. *Aethlon: The Journal of Sport Literature*, **25**(1), 241–251.

Douglas, K., & Carless, D. (2008d). Training or education? Negotiating a fuzzy line between what 'we' want and 'they' might need. *Annual Review of Golf Coaching 2008*, 1–13.

Douglas, K., & Carless, D. (2009a). Abandoning the performance narrative: Two women's stories of transition from professional golf. *Journal of Applied Sport Psychology*, **21**(2), 213–230.

Douglas, K., & Carless, D. (2009b). Exploring taboo issues in professional sport through a fictional approach. *Reflective Practice*, **10**(3), 311–323.

Douglas, K., & Carless, D. (2010). Restoring connections in physical activity and mental health research and practice: A confessional tale. *Qualitative Research in Sport and Exercise*, **2**(2).

Dowling Naess, F. (2001). Narratives about young men and masculinities in organised sport in Norway. *Sport, Education, and Society*, **6**, 125–142.

Eisner, E. (2008). Art and knowledge. In J. Knowles & A. Cole (Eds.), *Handbook of the Arts in Qualitative Research* (pp. 3–12). Thousand Oaks, CA: Sage.

Ellis, C., & Bochner, A. (2000). Autoethnography, personal narrative and reflexivity. In N. Denzin & Y. Lincoln (Eds.), *Handbook of Qualitative Research (second edition)* (pp. 733–768). Thousand Oaks, CA: Sage.

Ellis, N., Crone, D., Davey, R., & Grogan, S. (2007). Exercise interventions as an adjunct therapy for psychosis: A critical review. *British Journal of Clinical Psychology*, **46**, 95–111.

Etherington, K. (2003). (Ed.) *Trauma, the Body and Transformation: A Narrative Inquiry*. London: Jessica Kingsley.

Etherington, K. (2004). *Becoming a Reflexive Researcher*. London: Jessica-Kingsley.

Etherington, K. (2007a). Ethical research in reflexive relationships. *Qualitative Inquiry*, **13**(5), 599–616.

Etherington, K. (2007b). *Trauma, Drug Misuse and Transforming Identities: A Life Story Approach*. London: Jessica Kingsley.

Faulkner, G. (2005). Exercise as an adjunct treatment for schizophrenia. In: G. Faulkner, & A. Taylor (Eds.), *Exercise, Health and Mental Health: Emerging Relationships* (pp. 27–45). London: Routledge.

Faulkner, G., & Biddle, S. (1999). Exercise as an adjunct treatment for schizophrenia: A review of the literature. *Journal of Mental Health*, **8**(5), 441–457.

Faulkner, G., & Biddle, S. (2004). Exercise and depression: Considering variability and contextuality. *Journal of Sport and Exercise Psychology*, **26**(1), 3–18.

Faulkner, G., & Carless, D. (2006). Physical activity in the process of psychiatric rehabilitation: Theoretical and methodological issues. *Psychiatric Rehabilitation Journal*, **29**(4), 258–266.

Faulkner, G., & Sparkes, A. (1999). Exercise as therapy for schizophrenia: An ethnographic study. *Journal of Sport & Exercise Psychology*, **21**(1), 52–69.

Faulkner, G., & Taylor, A. (2005). *Exercise, Health and Mental Health: Emerging Relationships*. London: Routledge.

Fine, M., Weis, L., Weseen, S., & Wong, L. (2000). For whom? Qualitative research, representations, and social responsibilities. In N. Denzin & Y. Lincoln (Eds.), *Handbook of Qualitative Research (second edition)* (pp. 107–131). Thousand Oaks, CA: Sage.

Fogarty, M., & Happell, B. (2005). Exploring the benefits of an exercise program for people with schizophrenia: A qualitative study. *Issues in Mental Health Nursing*, **26**, 341–351.

Fox, K.R. (1999). The influence of physical activity on mental well-being. *Public Health Nutrition*, **2**, 411–18.

Fox, K.R. (2000). Physical activity and mental health: The natural partnership. *International Journal of Mental Health Promotion*, **2**(1), 4–12.

Frank, A. (1995). *The Wounded Storyteller*. Chicago: University of Chicago Press.

Frank, A. (2000a). The standpoint of storyteller. *Qualitative Health Research*, **10**(3), 354–365.

Frank, A. (2000b). Illness and autobiographical work: Dialogue as narrative destabilization. *Qualitative Sociology*, **23**(1), 135–156.

Frank, A. (2005). What is dialogical research and why should we do it? *Qualitative Health Research*, **15**(7), 964–974.

Gergen, K.J. (1999). *An Invitation to Social Constructionism*. Thousand Oaks, CA: Sage.

Gergen, M., & Gergen, K.J. (2006). Narratives in action. *Narrative Inquiry*, **16**(1), 112–121.

Gilligan, C. (1993). *In a Different Voice: Psychological Theory and Women's Development*. Cambridge, MA: Harvard University Press.

Grant, T. (Ed.) (2000). *Physical Activity and Mental Health: National Consensus Statements and Guidelines for Practitioners*. London: Health Education Authority.

Green, A., Patel, J., Goisman, R., Allison, D., & Blackburn, G. (2000). Weight gain from novel antipsychotic drugs: Need for action. *General Hospital Psychiatry*, **22**(4), 224–235.

Hayland, T. (1988). Values and health education: A critique of individualism. *Education Studies*, **14**, 23–21.

Holstein, J.A., & Gubrium, J.F. (2005). Interpretive practice and social action. In N. Denzin & Y. Lincoln (Eds.), *Handbook of Qualitative Research (third edition)* (pp. 483–505). Thousand Oaks, CA: Sage.

Ingham, A.G., Chase, M.A., & Butt, J. (2002). From the performance principle to the development principle: Every kid a winner? *Quest*, **54**, 308–331.

Janesick, V. (2000). The choreography of qualitative research: Minutes, improvisation and crystallisation. In N. Denzin & Y. Lincoln (Eds.), *Handbook of Qualitative Research (second edition)* (pp. 379–399). Thousand Oaks, CA: Sage.

Jones, M., & O'Beney, C. (2004). Promoting mental health through physical activity: Examples from practice. *Journal of Mental Health Promotion*, 3(1), 39–47.

Josselson, R. (1996). *The Space Between Us: Exploring the Dimensions of Human Relationships*. Thousand Oaks, CA: Sage.

Karp, D.A. (1996). *Speaking of Sadness*. New York, NY: Oxford University Press.

King, T. (2008). The art of indigenous knowledge: A million porcupines crying in the dark. In J. Knowles & A. Cole (Eds.), *Handbook of the Arts in Qualitative Research* (pp. 13–25). Thousand Oaks, CA: Sage.

Lawlor, D.A., & Hopker, S.W. (2001). The effectiveness of exercise as an intervention in the management of depression: Systematic review and meta-regression analysis of randomised controlled trials. *BMJ*, 322, 763.

Leith, L.M. (2002). *Foundations of Exercise and Mental Health*. Morgantown, WV: Fitness Information Technology.

Lieblich, A., Tuval-Mashiach, R., & Zilber, T. (1998). *Narrative Research: Reading, Analysis and Interpretation*. London: Sage.

Lysaker, P., & Lysaker, J. (2002). Narrative structure in psychosis: Schizophrenia and disruptions in the dialogical self. *Theory and Psychology*, 12(2), 207–220.

Lysaker, P., & Lysaker, J. (2006). A typology of narrative impoverishment in schizophrenia. *Counselling Psychology Quarterly*, 19(1), 57–68.

Madill, L., & Hopper, T. (2007). The best of the best discourse on health: Poetic insights on how professional sport socializes a family of men into hegemonic masculinity and physical inactivity. *American Journal of Men's Health*, 1(1), 44–59.

McAdams, D. (1993). *The Stories We Live By*. New York, NY: Guildford Press.

McAdams, D. (2001). *Coding autobiographical episodes for themes of agency and communication*. Retrieved from http://www.letus.org/foly/instruments/Agency_communion01.pdf

McDevitt, J., Snyder, M., Miller, A., & Wilbur, J. (2006). Perceptions of barriers and benefits to physical activity among outpatients in psychiatric rehabilitation. *Journal of Nursing Scholarship*, 38(1), 50–55.

McLeod, J. (1997). *Narrative and Psychotherapy*. London: Sage.

Miller, J.B. (1976). *Toward a New Psychology of Women*. Boston, MA: Beacon Press.

Morgan, W. (Ed.) (1997). *Physical Activity and Mental Health*. Washington, DC: Taylor & Francis.

Mutrie, N. (2000). The relationship between physical activity and clinically defined depression. In S. Biddle, K. Fox, & S. Boutcher (Eds.), *Physical Activity and Psychological Well-being* (pp. 46–62). London: Routledge.

Neilsen, L. (2008). Lyric inquiry. In J. Knowles & A. Cole (Eds.), *Handbook of the Arts in Qualitative Research* (pp. 93–102). Thousand Oaks, CA: Sage.

Nelson, M. (1994). *The Stronger Women Get, the More Men Love Football*. New York: Harcourt.

Nike/Youth Sport Trust (2006). *Girls in Sport Monitoring and Evaluation final report*. Loughborough, UK: Institute of Youth Sport.

Northcott, J. (2009). *Look Good Feel Great*. Poole, UK: Fitness First.

Ogilvie, B. (1997). Counselling for sports career termination. In J. May & M. Asken (Eds.), *Sport Psychology: The Psychological Health of the Athlete* (pp. 213–230). New York: PMA.

Ogilvie, B., & Howe, M. (1982). The trauma of termination from athletics. In J.M. Williams (Ed.), *Applied Sport Psychology: Personal Growth to Peak Performance* (pp. 365–382). Palo Alto, CA: Mayfield.

O'Neal, H., Dunn, A., & Martinsen, E. (2000). Depression and exercise. *International Journal of Sport Psychology*, **31**(2), 110–135.

Owens, C. (2004). The glass-walled asylum: A description of a lay residential community for the severely mentally ill. *Journal of Mental Health*, **13**(3), 319–332.

Patriksson, G. (1995). Scientific Review Part 2: The Significance of Sport for Society – Health, Socialisation, Economy. A scientific review prepared for the 8th conference of European Ministers responsible for sport, Lisbon, 17–18 May 1995, Council of Europe Press.

Pelias, R.J. (2004). *A Methodology of the Heart*. Walnut Creek, CA: AltaMira Press.

Raine, P., Truman, C., & Southerst, A. (2002). The development of a community gym for people with mental health problems: Influences on psychological accessibility. *Journal of Mental Health* **11**(1), 43–53.

Rees, T., & Hardy, L. (2000). An investigation of the social support experiences of high-level sports performers. *Sports Psychologist*, **14**, 327–347.

Rees, T., Smith, B., & Sparkes, A. (2003). The influence of social support on the lived experiences of spinal cord injured sportsmen. *Sports Psychologist*, **17**, 135–156.

Repper, J., & Perkins, R. (2003). *Social Inclusion and Recovery*. Edinburgh, Baillière Tindall.

Richardson, C., Faulkner, G., McDevitt, J., Skrinar, G., Hutchinson, D., & Piette, J. (2005). Integrating physical activity into mental health services for individuals with serious mental illness. *Psychiatric Services*, **56**, 324–331.

Richardson, L. (2000). Writing: A method of inquiry. In N. Denzin & Y. Lincoln (Eds.), *Handbook of Qualitative Research (second edition)* (pp. 923–948). Thousand Oaks, CA: Sage.

Riessman, C.K. (2008). *Narrative Methods for the Human Sciences*. Thousand Oaks, CA: Sage.

Rogers, A., & Pilgrim, D. (2005). *A Sociology of Mental Health and Illness (third edition)*. Maidenhead, UK: Open University Press.

Rudacille, D. (2006). *The Riddle of Gender*. New York: Anchor Books.

Saxena, S., Van Ommeren, M., Tang, K., & Armstrong, T. (2005). Mental health benefits of physical activity. *Journal of Mental Health*, **14**(5), 445–451.

Scheibe, K. (1986). Self-narratives and adventure. In T. Sarbin (Ed.), *Narrative Psychology: The Storied Nature of Human Conduct* (pp. 129–151). New York: Prager.

Shilling, C. (2005). *The Body in Culture, Technology and Society*. Sage: London.

Shilling, C., & Bunsell, T. (2009). The female bodybuilder as a gender outlaw. *Qualitative Research in Sport and Exercise*, **1**(2), 125–159.

Sinclair, D., & Orlick, T. (1993). Positive transitions from high-performance sport. *Sport Psychologist*, **7**, 138–150.

Skrinar, G., Huxley, N., Hutchinson, D., Menninger, E., & Glew, P. (2005). The role of a fitness intervention on people with serious psychiatric disabilities. *Psychiatric Rehabilitation Journal*, **29**(2), 122–127.

Smith, B. (1999). The Abyss: Exploring depression through a narrative of the self. *Qualitative Inquiry*, **5**(2), 264–279.

Smith, B. (2010). Narrative inquiry: Ongoing conversations and questions for sport and exercise psychology research. *International Review of Sport and Exercise Psychology*, **3**(1), 87–107.

Smith, B., & Sparkes, A.C. (2002). Men, sport, spinal cord injury, and the construction of coherence: Narrative practice in action. *Qualitative Research*, **2**(2), 143–171.

Smith, B., & Sparkes, A.C. (2004). Men, sport, and spinal cord injury: An analysis of metaphors and narrative types. *Disability and Society*, **19**(6), 509–612.

Smith, B., & Sparkes, A.C. (2005). Analyzing talk in qualitative inquiry: Exploring possibilities, problems, and tensions. *Quest*, **57**(2), 213–242.

Smith, B., & Sparkes, A.C. (2006). Narrative inquiry in psychology: Exploring the tensions within. *Qualitative Research in Psychology*, **3**(3), 169–192.

Smith, B., & Sparkes, A.C. (2009). Narrative analysis and sport and exercise psychology: Understanding stories in diverse ways. *Psychology of Sport and Exercise*, **10**(2), 279–288.

Soundy, A., Faulkner, G., & Taylor, A. (2007). Exploring variability and perceptions of lifestyle activity among individuals with severe and enduring mental health problems: A qualitative study. *Journal of Mental Health*, **16**(4), 493–503.

Sparkes, A.C. (1992). The paradigms debate: An extended review and celebration of difference. In A. Sparkes (Ed.), *Research in Physical Education and Sport: Exploring Alternative Visions* (pp. 9–60). London: Falmer Press.

Sparkes, A.C. (1996). The fatal flaw. *Qualitative Inquiry*, **2**(4), 463–494.

Sparkes, A.C. (1997). Reflections on the socially constructed physical self. In K. Fox (Ed.), *The Physical Self* (pp. 83–110). Champaign, IL: Human Kinetics.

Sparkes, A.C. (1998). Athletic identity: An Achilles heel to the survival of the self. *Qualitative Health Research*, **8**(5), 644–664.

Sparkes, A.C. (2000). Autoethnographies and narratives of self. *Sociology of Sport Journal*, **17**(1), 21–43.

Sparkes, A.C. (2002). *Telling Tales in Sport and Physical Activity*. Champaign, IL: Human Kinetics.

Sparkes, A.C. (2005). Narrative analysis: Exploring the *whats* and the *hows* of personal stories. In: M. Holloway (Ed.), *Qualitative Research in Health Care* (pp. 91–209). Maidenhead, UK: Open University Press.

Sparkes, A.C. (2007). Embodiment, academics, and the audit culture: A story seeking consideration. *Qualitative Research*, **7**(4), 521–550.

Sparkes, A.C. (2008). Sport and physical education: embracing new forms of representation. In: J. Knowles & A. Cole (Eds.), *Handbook of the Arts in Qualitative Research* (pp. 653–664). Thousand Oaks, CA: Sage.

Sparkes, A.C. (2009). Ethnography and the senses: Challenges and possibilities. *Qualitative Research in Sport and Exercise*, **1**(1), 21–35.

Sparkes, A.C., & Douglas, K. (2007). Making the case for poetic representations: An example in action. *Sport Psychologist*, **21**(2), 170–189.

Sparkes, A.C., & Smith, B. (2003). Men, sport, spinal cord injury and narrative time. *Qualitative Research*, 3(3), 295–320.

Sparkes, A.C., & Smith, B. (2008). Narrative constructionist inquiry. In J. Holstein & J. Gubrium (Eds.), *Handbook of Constructionist Research* (pp. 295–314). London: Guilford Press.

Stathopolou, G., Powers, M., Berry, A., Smits, J., & Otto, M. (2006). Exercise interventions for mental health: A quantitative and qualitative review. *Clinical Psychology – Science and Practice* 13(2), 179–193.

Stone, B. (2004). Towards a writing without power: Notes on the narration of madness. *Auto/Biography*, **12**, 16–33.

Stone, B. (2006). Diaries, self-talk, and psychosis: Writing as a place to live. *Auto/Biography*, **14**, 41–58.

Stone, B. (2009). Running man. *Qualitative Research in Sport and Exercise*, 1(1), 67–71.

Svoboda, B., & Vanek, M. (1982). Retirement from high-level competition. In T. Orlick, J. Partington, & J. Salmela (Eds.), *Mental Training for Coaches and Athletes* (pp. 166–175). Ottawa: Coaching Association of Canada.

Teychenne, M., Ball, K., & Salmon, J. (2008a). Physical activity and likelihood of depression in adults: A review. *Preventive Medicine*, **46**, 397–411.

Teychenne, M., Ball, K., & Salmon, J. (2008b). Associations between physical activity and depressive symptoms in women. *International Journal of Behavioral Nutrition and Physical Activity*, **5**: 27.

UK Sport (2006). *Progress Made Towards Objectives and Targets Set for 2005 and Analysis of the Current Situation*. London: UK Sport.

US Department of Health and Human Services (1999). *Mental Health: A Report of the Surgeon General*. Rockville, MD: US DHHS.

US Department of Health and Human Services (n.d.). Downloaded from http://mentalhealth.samhsa.gov/features/hp2010/terminology.asp on 14 October 2006.

Van Maanen, J. (1988). *Tales of the Field*. Chicago, University of Chicago Press.

Van Raalte, J., & Anderson, M. (2007). When sport psychology consulting is a means to an end(ing): Roles and agendas when helping athletes leave their sports. *Sport Psychologist*, **21**, 227–242.

White, M., & Epston, D. (1990). *Narrative Means to Therapeutic Ends*. New York: Norton.

Wolcott, H.F. (1994). *Transforming Qualitative Data*. Thousand Oaks, CA: Sage.

Women's Sports Foundation (2005). *Physical Activity in Older Women in Cornwall*. London: Women's Sports Foundation.

Zanker, C., & Gard, M. (2008). Fatness, fitness, and the moral universe of sport and physical activity. *Sociology of Sport Journal*, **25**, 48–65.

Index